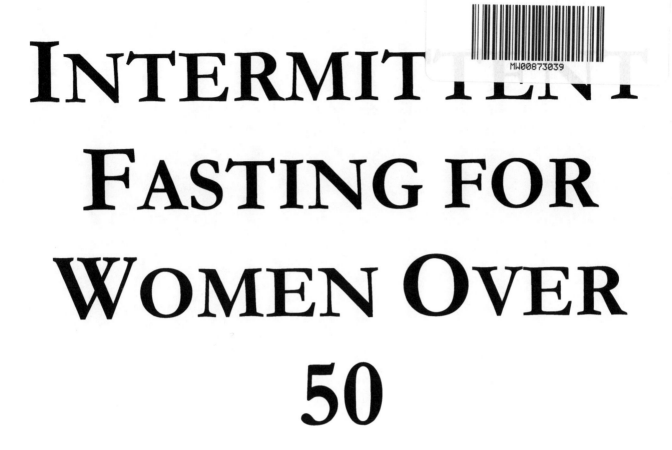

INTERMITTENT FASTING FOR WOMEN OVER 50

Rejuvenate Your Life with Science-Backed Fasting Techniques and Delectable Dishes Tailored for Vibrant Health

Addison Sturgeon

TABLE OF CONTENTS

CHAPTER 1: INTRODUCTION TO INTERMITTENT FASTING FOR WOMEN OVER 50

As we gracefully journey beyond the threshold of 50, the landscape of our bodies and needs transforms, ushering in a period where wisdom meets the necessity for adaptability in health practices. One such adaptable method that has emerged as particularly beneficial is intermittent fasting—a concept that might seem daunting at first but reveals itself as a rejuvenating partner through the later stages of life.

Intermittent fasting isn't just another diet fad; it's a time-tested practice backed by science, which helps in recalibrating the body's metabolic processes and enhancing overall well-being. Especially for women over 50, this approach addresses the nuanced shifts in hormonal balances and metabolic rates that often accompany menopause and the aging process. The beauty of intermittent fasting lies in its flexibility, which allows you to tailor your eating patterns to fit your lifestyle while still reaping significant health benefits.

But why does intermittent fasting resonate so well with women in their golden years? The answer lies in its simplicity and the profound impact it has on the body's cellular functions. By alternating between periods of eating and fasting, the body learns to optimize energy use from fat stores, reducing inflammation and improving metabolic health. This isn't just about weight loss—though it is often a welcome benefit—it's about setting a foundation for a vibrant later life, enhancing everything from cognitive function to cardiovascular health.

Moreover, intermittent fasting serves as a gateway to mindfulness about food and health, encouraging a deeper connection to how we nourish our bodies. It's about making intentional choices, not restrictive ones, allowing for a diet that includes all food groups but honors the timing of intake to optimize health benefits.

Embracing intermittent fasting as you age is like tuning a musical instrument; it's about finding the right rhythm that brings harmony to your body and life. As we delve deeper into this chapter, we will explore the various methods of intermittent fasting, understand the science behind its effectiveness, and learn how to integrate it seamlessly into our lives—ensuring that the journey through our fifties and beyond is not just about surviving, but thriving.

1.1 WHAT IS INTERMITTENT FASTING AND WHY IT WORKS FOR WOMEN OVER 50

Intermittent fasting is like the rhythm of the ocean; it's about cycles and patterns, ebb and flow. It's not simply a diet but a way of life that aligns our eating patterns with our body's natural instincts and scientific principles. At its core, intermittent fasting involves alternating periods of eating and fasting, which not only helps manage weight but also enhances metabolic health and cellular repair. As women over 50, this practice holds particular promise, not just for its physical benefits but for its potential to rejuvenate and reset our biological clocks.

For many women, the years post-50 brings about a host of changes. Hormonal shifts, particularly due to menopause, can make it harder to maintain muscle mass and keep off excess weight. Metabolism slows, and the risk of chronic diseases such as type 2 diabetes and cardiovascular issues inches upward. It's during this pivotal time that intermittent fasting can step in as a powerful tool. By harnessing the body's natural response to fasting, this practice helps improve insulin sensitivity, decrease inflammation, and enhance brain function.

The Science Behind Fasting

The concept of intermittent fasting is rooted in evolutionary science. Historically, humans didn't have access to the constant food supply we enjoy today. Our ancestors often went through periods of feast and famine, and as a result, our bodies evolved to perform optimally with intermittent periods of not eating. During fasting periods, significant hormonal changes occur in the body. Levels of insulin drop, facilitating fat burning. Human growth hormone (HGH) levels increase, which are crucial for metabolic health and muscle strength—two critical concerns for aging women.

Moreover, fasting triggers a cellular response known as autophagy, where cells begin to clean out damaged components. This process, which won the Nobel Prize in Physiology or Medicine in 2016 for its researcher, Dr. Yoshinori Ohsumi, is particularly beneficial as it promotes cellular repair and can have anti-aging effects, something incredibly beneficial for women dealing with the cellular decline associated with aging.

Why It Appeals to Women Over 50

For women over 50, the appeal of intermittent fasting is multifaceted. Firstly, it offers a way to manage weight more effectively at a time when many women find shedding pounds more challenging. The hormonal changes of menopause, including decreased estrogen levels, often lead to increased abdominal fat, a risk factor for heart disease and diabetes. Intermittent fasting helps by improving metabolic flexibility—the body's ability to switch between burning carbs and fats for energy—which often gets sluggish as we age.

Secondly, intermittent fasting improves other markers of health that are particularly pertinent as we grow older. It reduces inflammation, a key driver of many chronic diseases, and improves blood sugar control. Additionally, it increases levels of brain-derived neurotrophic factor (BDNF), a protein that supports brain health and can protect against Alzheimer's disease and other forms of cognitive decline.

Personalizing Fasting for Women Over 50

While the benefits are clear, the approach to intermittent fasting should be personalized, especially for women at midlife and beyond. There are several popular methods of intermittent fasting, including the 16/8 method, where you fast for 16 hours and eat within an 8-hour window; the 5:2 method, which involves eating normally for five days of the week while restricting calories to about 500-600 for the other two days; and 'Eat-Stop-Eat', which might involve a 24-hour fast once or twice a week.

The choice of method depends on one's lifestyle, health status, and goals. For many women, a gentle start with the 16/8 method proves less daunting and more manageable. It's crucial to consider how each method fits into your daily life and how it makes you feel. Listening to your body is key; if a particular fasting schedule leads to feelings of extreme discomfort or disrupts sleep, adjustments are necessary. This flexibility is what makes intermittent fasting sustainable and effective, rather than being another strict diet regime.

Implementing Intermittent Fasting

Starting intermittent fasting involves more than choosing when to eat and when to fast. It's about integrating this pattern into your life in a way that feels natural and sustainable. Begin slowly, perhaps by delaying breakfast to shorten the eating window and gradually increase the fasting period. It's also essential to focus on nutritious foods during eating periods to ensure your body gets the necessary nutrients to thrive.

Hydration plays a crucial role as well. During fasting periods, ensure you drink plenty of water. Herbal teas are also a great option as they can be soothing and don't break the fast.

Lastly, it's vital to monitor your health throughout the process. Regular check-ups with a healthcare provider can help track blood markers and other health indicators to ensure the fasting regimen is beneficial.

Intermittent fasting holds a powerful potential to transform health, particularly for women over 50 who face unique health challenges. By understanding and implementing this ancient yet scientifically supported practice, you can tap into profound benefits that extend far beyond weight loss, enriching your later years with vigor and vitality. As we continue to explore intermittent fasting in this chapter, remember that this is not just about dieting—it's about rediscovering a rhythm of eating that aligns with our deepest biological principles and health goals.

1.2 DIFFERENT TYPES OF INTERMITTENT FASTING METHODS

In the evolving narrative of health and wellness for women over 50, intermittent fasting stands out not just as a singular approach, but as a palette of diverse methods, each with its own rhythm and cadence. This versatility in fasting techniques allows it to be woven seamlessly into the fabric of our daily lives, respecting our unique schedules, preferences, and health requirements. As we explore the various intermittent fasting methods, imagine each as a different path in a garden, inviting you to walk it and discover the one that aligns best with your lifestyle and health goals.

The 16/8 Method

One of the most popular and accessible forms of intermittent fasting is the 16/8 method, also known as time-restricted eating. Here, the fasting period spans 16 hours, which for many might include the hours spent sleeping. The remaining 8 hours form the eating window. This method is particularly appealing for its simplicity and ease of integration into daily routines. For example, if you finish your evening meal by 8 p.m., your next meal would be at noon the following day. This method not only helps regulate the body's insulin levels but also aligns with natural circadian rhythms, supporting metabolic and hormonal balance — crucial elements for women navigating the post-menopausal phase.

The 5:2 Diet

Another approach is the 5:2 diet, where you eat normally for five days of the week and reduce calorie intake on the other two days to about 500-600 calories per day. This method allows a degree of flexibility that can be less daunting, making it a good option for those who may find daily fasting too restrictive. It encourages a sense of dietary freedom while still promoting significant health benefits such as improved blood sugar levels and reduced inflammation. The 5:2 method also taps into the body's ability to use fat as fuel on low-calorie days, which can be an effective strategy for weight management and metabolic health.

Eat-Stop-Eat

For those who might be looking for a more intensive fasting experience, the Eat-Stop-Eat method involves a full 24-hour fast once or twice a week. This could mean not eating from dinner one day until dinner the next day. While it offers profound health benefits, including enhanced autophagy and reduced caloric intake, it requires a good deal of mental resilience and preparation. It's important for anyone considering this method to ease into it slowly and consult with a healthcare provider, especially to ensure it doesn't disrupt essential nutrient intake or overall health.

The Warrior Diet

The Warrior Diet is another intriguing method, where fasting and feeding are divided into 20-hour fasts and 4-hour eating windows. During the 20-hour period, light snacking on raw fruits and vegetables is allowed, leading up to one large, nutritious meal in the evening. This diet draws on the ancient idea of warriors who ate little during the day and feasted at night. It can be particularly beneficial for those looking to improve their diet quality by focusing on a substantial, nutrient-dense meal that provides all the necessary dietary components within a concentrated eating window.

Alternative Day Fasting

Alternating between fasting days and eating days is the cornerstone of Alternate-Day Fasting. This method can be quite flexible — some versions allow for about 500 calories during fasting days, while others recommend no caloric intake at all. Alternate-Day Fasting can be particularly effective for weight loss and improving cardiovascular health. However, it's essential to approach this method with care, ensuring that on eating days, the food consumed provides a rich array of nutrients to support overall health and well-being.

Customizing Your Approach

Choosing the right intermittent fasting method is akin to choosing a dance partner; it needs to match your rhythm and pace. It's important to consider not only your health goals but also your lifestyle. For many women over 50, the flexibility of the fasting schedule is key to its sustainability and effectiveness. Factors like sleep patterns, daily activities, and energy needs should all be considered when selecting the appropriate fasting method.

Moreover, it's crucial to listen to your body's cues. Effective fasting should feel challenging yet invigorating. If a method leads to prolonged fatigue, irritability, or other distressing symptoms, it may not be the right fit. Adapting the method to suit individual health conditions, preferences, and responses is perfectly acceptable. Remember, intermittent fasting is not about deprivation; it's about empowering yourself to make health decisions that rejuvenate and sustain.

Exploring these various intermittent fasting methods offers a canvas on which to paint your nutritional strategy. Each method has its merits and challenges, but all share a common goal: to enhance your health by aligning eating patterns with the body's natural rhythms and needs. As you consider these options, think of them as tools in your health toolkit, each capable of sculpting a more vibrant, energized version of yourself in the golden years of life. Choosing the right tool is just the beginning of a transformative journey toward rejuvenated health and vitality.

1.3 SETTING REALISTIC GOALS AND EXPECTATIONS

Embarking on the journey of intermittent fasting, especially for women over 50, is akin to setting sail on a vast ocean. The path can be exhilarating and challenging, filled with discoveries and necessary adjustments. As with any expedition, the success often hinges on setting realistic goals and maintaining proper expectations. This isn't just about transforming your diet; it's about changing your lifestyle in a way that fosters health and vitality as you age.

Understanding the Realistic Outcomes of Intermittent Fasting

Intermittent fasting offers numerous health benefits, such as improved metabolic rates, reduced inflammation, and enhanced brain function. However, the results can vary based on individual health backgrounds, lifestyles, and commitment. For women over 50, it's crucial to recognize that changes in body composition and metabolism due to menopause can affect how quickly and effectively these benefits manifest.

It's common to hear about rapid weight loss and transformative health changes from fasting, but it's essential to approach these narratives with a balanced perspective. Weight loss, for example, should be gradual. A drop of about 1-2 pounds per week is considered healthy and sustainable. Rapid weight loss is often hard to maintain and can strip the body of essential nutrients, leading to other health issues.

Setting Goals That Resonate with Personal Health Needs

When setting goals, consider what is most important for your health and well-being. Are you focusing on losing weight, improving blood sugar levels, enhancing cognitive function, or perhaps all three? Goals should be S.M.A.R.T (Specific, Measurable, Achievable, Relevant, and Time-bound). For instance, instead of aiming to "lose weight," a more specific goal would be to "lose 10 pounds in the next three months by practicing the 16/8 intermittent fasting method."

Furthermore, it's vital to tailor your goals to your current health conditions. If you have pre-existing health issues like diabetes or high blood pressure, adjustments may be needed, and consulting with healthcare professionals becomes essential. These professionals can provide valuable insights and periodic assessments to ensure your fasting regimen complements your health needs without causing adverse effects.

Adjusting Expectations to Fit Individual Lifestyles

Every woman's lifestyle is different, influencing how effectively intermittent fasting can be integrated. For someone with a highly active social life, for instance, fasting methods requiring long periods without eating might seem daunting and impractical. In such cases, a more flexible approach, like the 5:2 method, might be more suitable as it allows for normal eating on most days.

It's also crucial to consider the emotional and psychological impacts of fasting. Feeling irritable or overly stressed during fasting periods is a sign that adjustments might be necessary. Emotional well-being is as important as physical health, and your fasting regimen should not be a source of significant stress or discomfort.

Embracing a Holistic View of Progress

Progress in intermittent fasting isn't just measured by the scale or the fit of your clothes; it also includes improvements in energy levels, mental clarity, and overall vitality. These aspects are sometimes overlooked when expectations are narrowly focused on weight loss. Keep a journal to document not only your dietary intake and fasting hours but also how you feel physically and emotionally. This holistic view of progress can provide a more comprehensive understanding of how intermittent fasting is influencing your life.

Patience and Perseverance: Key Virtues

Patience is a virtue, especially when adapting to a new eating pattern like intermittent fasting. The body needs time to adjust to changes in meal timing and frequency. Initial side effects, such as mild headaches or temporary energy dips, are common as the body transitions from glucose to fat as its primary energy source. Perseverance is crucial during this phase. The benefits of intermittent fasting often become more apparent and pronounced after the body has fully adapted to the new routine, which can take several weeks or even months.

Setting realistic goals and expectations is the cornerstone of a successful intermittent fasting plan, especially for women over 50. By understanding the potential benefits and challenges, tailoring goals to individual needs, and maintaining a balanced perspective on progress, you can ensure that your fasting journey is not only successful but also enriching. Remember, intermittent fasting is more than a path to weight loss; it's a journey towards a healthier, more vibrant version of yourself. As you move forward, allow yourself the flexibility to adapt and the grace to accept the ebbs and flows of this transformative experience.

CHAPTER 2: BENEFITS OF INTERMITTENT FASTING FOR AGING WOMEN

As we gracefully embrace the golden years of life, the pursuit of health and vitality becomes a paramount concern. For women navigating the complexities of aging, intermittent fasting emerges not merely as a dietary trend, but as a profound ally in enhancing wellness and extending quality of life. This chapter delves into the myriad benefits that intermittent fasting offers specifically to aging women, exploring how this time-honored practice supports both body and mind amidst the changes that accompany the later stages of life.

Intermittent fasting, with its diverse approaches, aligns beautifully with the body's natural rhythms, encouraging a host of beneficial effects. These benefits extend beyond the commonly sought-after weight management, reaching into the very essence of what it means to age healthily. It enhances metabolic health, supports hormonal balance, and offers promising implications for longevity and disease prevention. Each of these benefits addresses the unique challenges faced by women over fifty, such as the metabolic slowdown and hormonal shifts that mark menopause and beyond.

Moreover, intermittent fasting does more than just address physical health. It also plays a crucial role in mental clarity and emotional well-being, fostering a sense of control and empowerment over one's health decisions. This empowerment is a vital component of the journey, as it transforms the experience of aging into one of renewal and positivity.

In this chapter, we will weave through the scientific insights and personal stories that illuminate how intermittent fasting can be a cornerstone of vibrant health for aging women. Through a tapestry of research and real-life experiences, the narrative will reveal not just why intermittent fasting works, but how it can be a source of rejuvenation, a ritual of self-care, and a pathway to thriving in the years that many call the best of their lives.

2.1 METABOLIC HEALTH AND WEIGHT MANAGEMENT

In the journey through midlife and beyond, women face unique metabolic challenges, primarily driven by hormonal changes and a natural decline in metabolic rate. However, amidst these inevitable shifts, intermittent fasting emerges as a beacon of hope, a strategy not just for weight management but also for enhancing overall metabolic health.

The Metabolic Shift

As women enter their fifties and beyond, the body undergoes significant transformations. Estrogen levels decline, which can lead to a decrease in metabolic rate and an increase in abdominal fat. This fat is not just a cosmetic concern but a health risk, associated with higher chances of developing heart disease, type 2 diabetes, and other metabolic syndromes. Herein lies the first benefit of intermittent fasting: by improving insulin sensitivity and increasing growth hormone levels, it helps combat these metabolic slowdowns and redistributes body fat away from the midsection.

Intermittent Fasting and Insulin Sensitivity

One of the key mechanisms through which intermittent fasting boosts metabolic health is by enhancing insulin sensitivity. During the fasting periods, the body reduces its insulin production due to lowered food intake. This reduction allows the cells to become more sensitive to insulin when it is produced, a stark contrast to the insulin resistance often seen in older adults, especially post-menopausal women. Enhanced insulin sensitivity means that the body is better able to utilize glucose from the bloodstream, leading to better blood sugar control and reduced fat storage.

Growth Hormone: The Anti-Aging Ally

Intermittent fasting has been shown to increase levels of human growth hormone (HGH), sometimes referred to as the anti-aging hormone. HGH plays a crucial role in maintaining muscle mass, which naturally declines with age. This decline in muscle mass contributes to a slower metabolic rate, making weight loss and maintenance more challenging. By boosting HGH levels, intermittent fasting not only helps preserve muscle mass but also aids in burning fat more effectively, thereby supporting healthy aging.

The Practicality of Weight Management

Weight management in later life can often seem like a frustrating puzzle. However, intermittent fasting offers a practical solution that does not require drastic dietary changes. By simply altering 'when' rather than 'what' you eat, it can lead to a natural reduction in calorie intake. Many women find this method less daunting than traditional diets that require constant calorie counting and restrictive eating plans. The flexibility of intermittent fasting allows it to be adapted to different lifestyles, making it a sustainable approach to weight management.

Autophagy: Cellular Cleansing

Another significant aspect of intermittent fasting is its ability to initiate autophagy, a process where cells remove toxins, repair damage, and recycle parts that are no longer functional. This cellular cleansing process is crucial for preventing diseases that are often associated with aging, such as Alzheimer's and other forms of dementia, as well as for maintaining overall cellular health. The enhanced autophagy from intermittent fasting can thus play a pivotal role in extending life expectancy and improving quality of life.

The Synergistic Effects on Metabolism

Beyond individual benefits, intermittent fasting creates a synergistic effect on the body's metabolism. It enhances the efficiency of energy use, reduces oxidative stress, and improves fat oxidation. These effects are particularly beneficial for women over 50, who may be battling sluggish metabolisms and increased oxidative stress levels due to aging. Intermittent fasting helps reset the metabolic machinery, giving the body a chance to regain its balance and function optimally.

Long-Term Sustainability

Adopting intermittent fasting is not just about the short-term benefits; it's about creating a long-term sustainable practice. For many aging women, this means finding a rhythm with fasting that respects their body's needs and lifestyle preferences. The process involves trial and adjustment, listening carefully to the body's responses, and being open to modifying fasting schedules as needed. The goal is to create a way of eating that feels natural, manageable, and beneficial across various stages of life.

The relationship between intermittent fasting, metabolic health, and weight management is a powerful one, offering aging women a tool not just for maintaining physical health but also for enhancing their overall life quality. By understanding and implementing intermittent fasting, women can take an active role in managing their metabolism, embracing a practice that supports their body's changing needs while fostering resilience against age-related declines. This approach does not promise a quick fix but offers a pathway to a healthier, more vibrant life through mindful, intentional eating patterns.

2.2 HORMONAL BALANCE AND MENOPAUSAL SUPPORT

Navigating the turbulent waters of menopause presents a significant challenge for many women as they enter their golden years. Hormonal fluctuations can disrupt not just physical health but emotional well-being. Amidst this storm, intermittent fasting emerges as a guiding light, offering not just a beacon of hope for managing weight but as a significant ally in stabilizing hormonal balance and easing menopausal symptoms.

The Impact of Menopause on Hormonal Health

Menopause is marked by the end of a woman's reproductive years, accompanied by a decline in estrogen and progesterone levels. This hormonal upheaval can lead to various symptoms like hot flashes, night sweats, mood swings, and increased anxiety, which can affect the quality of life. Beyond discomfort, these hormonal changes increase the risk of developing osteoporosis and cardiovascular disease, making management crucial during this time.

How Intermittent Fasting Plays a Role

Intermittent fasting can influence hormonal health through several mechanisms. One of the most significant impacts is on insulin sensitivity. As mentioned, fasting improves how the body's cells respond to insulin, reducing the risk of insulin resistance, which is commonly exacerbated during menopause. Better insulin management helps moderate the body's hormone levels, including those critical for women's health like estrogen and progesterone.

Support for Adrenal Glands

Stress plays a crucial role in hormonal balance, with cortisol, the stress hormone, having a profound effect. The adrenal glands, which produce cortisol, are already under pressure to compensate for the lower production of estrogen and progesterone during menopause. Intermittent fasting can help support adrenal function by normalizing cortisol levels and reducing oxidative stress, thus alleviating some menopausal symptoms and contributing to overall hormonal balance.

Enhancing Growth Hormone Production

The benefits of increased human growth hormone (HGH) production through intermittent fasting are particularly valuable during menopause. HGH helps maintain muscle mass, which tends to decline with age and hormonal changes. By improving muscle mass and strength, HGH not only enhances metabolic health but also supports skeletal health, reducing the risk of osteoporosis, which becomes a significant concern post-menopause.

Autophagy and Cellular Health

Autophagy, the body's way of cleaning out damaged cells and regenerating new ones, is another critical benefit of intermittent fasting that supports hormonal balance. This process helps remove estrogen receptors that may become dysfunctional and contribute to estrogen dominance, a common issue during the perimenopausal period. By promoting healthier cell function, intermittent fasting helps ensure that hormone receptors and the enzymes responsible for hormone metabolism function optimally, supporting overall hormonal health.

Modulating the Thyroid Axis

Intermittent fasting also impacts thyroid function, which is intricately linked to estrogen. The thyroid plays a pivotal role in regulating metabolism, energy levels, and body temperature—all areas that can be problematic during menopause. Fasting has been shown to help modulate thyroid activity, which can help alleviate some symptoms associated with menopausal changes, such as fluctuations in body weight and energy levels.

Psychological Benefits and Emotional Well-being

Beyond the physical aspects, intermittent fasting can also have psychological benefits, improving mood and cognitive function. The practice can increase brain-derived neurotrophic factor (BDNF), a protein that plays a significant role in emotional health and cognitive function. Increased BDNF can help counteract mood swings and cognitive decline associated with hormonal changes during menopause.

Practical Considerations for Implementing Fasting During Menopause

Adopting intermittent fasting during menopause requires consideration of individual health needs and symptoms. It is crucial to start slowly, possibly with milder fasting protocols like the 14/10 or 16/8 method, and to consult healthcare providers to ensure the approach is safe and effective given one's specific health profile. Staying hydrated, ensuring a nutrient-dense diet during eating windows, and closely monitoring how the body responds to the changes are essential steps to maximizing the benefits while minimizing potential stressors or negative impacts.

Intermittent fasting offers a promising approach to managing the complex changes associated with menopause. By supporting hormonal balance, enhancing metabolic health, and improving emotional well-being, this practice can significantly ease the transition through menopause and help women maintain a vibrant, healthy lifestyle in their later years. As each woman's journey through menopause is unique, so too should be their approach to intermittent fasting, tailored to fit their specific health needs and lifestyle preferences.

2.3 LONGEVITY AND DISEASE PREVENTION

The golden years of life are often anticipated with a mix of excitement and apprehension, as aging can bring about not just wisdom and leisure but also an increased risk of chronic diseases. Yet, what if there was a way to turn the tide on aging, extending not just the number of years we live but also enhancing the quality of those years? Intermittent fasting offers just that—a beacon of hope not only for prolonging life but also for fortifying it against many diseases that threaten it.

The Link Between Intermittent Fasting, Longevity, and Disease Prevention

At its core, intermittent fasting affects the body at a molecular and cellular level, influencing everything from metabolic pathways to hormone levels, which play pivotal roles in health and aging. The practice has been linked to longevity primarily through its ability to improve metabolic efficiency and overall body composition, but the benefits extend much deeper.

Autophagy: The Body's Own Anti-Aging Mechanism

One of the most significant ways intermittent fasting contributes to longevity is through autophagy, a process that helps repair damaged cells and recycle proteins that are no longer effective. Autophagy is essentially the body's way of cleaning up accumulated cellular debris, which, if left unchecked, can lead to cellular dysfunction and disease. Enhancing autophagy can help prevent diseases associated with aging such as Alzheimer's, Parkinson's, and other neurodegenerative disorders by maintaining cellular health and function.

Reducing Inflammation: A Key to Preventing Chronic Diseases

Chronic inflammation is a common thread linking many age-related diseases, including heart disease, diabetes, and cancer. Intermittent fasting has been shown to reduce markers of inflammation, which may help decrease the risk of these conditions. This reduction in inflammation is partly attributed to the decrease in fat mass that often accompanies fasting, as adipose tissue contributes to inflammatory processes in the body.

Impact on Cardiovascular Health

Heart disease remains the leading cause of death worldwide, and its prevalence increases with age. Intermittent fasting positively affects several key risk factors for cardiovascular disease, including blood pressure, cholesterol levels, and triglycerides. Fasting can improve the lipid profile by increasing HDL (good) cholesterol and decreasing LDL (bad) cholesterol and triglycerides, thereby reducing the risk of atherosclerosis, heart attacks, and strokes.

Enhancing Brain Health and Function

The benefits of intermittent fasting also extend to cognitive function and neurological health. Fasting increases the production of brain-derived neurotrophic factor (BDNF), a protein that supports the survival of existing neurons and encourages the growth of new neurons and synapses. High levels of BDNF can protect against Alzheimer's disease and depression, which are more prevalent in older adults. Additionally, fasting can enhance the brain's resistance to stress and injury, further supporting cognitive health and function.

Regulating Hormonal Balance

Hormones have a profound impact on the aging process, influencing everything from energy metabolism to brain function. Intermittent fasting helps to optimize the levels of key hormones, including insulin, human growth hormone, and leptin, which can help maintain youthfulness and vitality. By improving insulin sensitivity, fasting reduces the risk of type 2 diabetes, a common age-related condition. Additionally, increased levels of growth hormone contribute to muscle strength and mass, which typically decline with age.

Cancer Prevention and Intermittent Fasting

Emerging research suggests that intermittent fasting may also play a role in cancer prevention. By reducing inflammation, improving immune function, and lowering blood sugar levels, fasting creates a less favorable environment for cancer cells to thrive. Furthermore, fasting can enhance the effectiveness of chemotherapy by making cancer cells more susceptible to treatment while protecting normal cells.

Building a Sustainable Practice

Adopting intermittent fasting for longevity and disease prevention is about more than just skipping meals; it's about creating a sustainable, healthy lifestyle that includes regular physical activity, adequate sleep, and a diet rich in nutrients. For women over 50, it's crucial to approach fasting with a focus on gradual, manageable changes that can be maintained over the long term, ensuring that the practice contributes positively to both longevity and quality of life.

Integrating intermittent fasting into one's lifestyle offers a powerful tool for aging gracefully and healthily. It empowers women over 50 to take proactive steps toward disease prevention and longevity by leveraging the body's natural mechanisms for maintaining health. As we explore these profound benefits, intermittent fasting reveals itself not just as a dietary pattern but as a pathway to a revitalized life, filled with vitality and resilience against the diseases of aging. Through understanding and applying this practice, aging can be faced not with fear but with confidence and grace.

DOWNLOAD YOUR BONUS

The Healthy Juicing Collection

Dear Reader,

Thank you for purchasing this book and downloading the bonus content.

Your support means the world to me. I hope you find value in the insights and stories shared within these pages.

If you enjoyed the book, I would be incredibly grateful if you could take a moment to leave a review on Amazon. Your feedback helps me improve and reach more readers like you.

Warm regards,

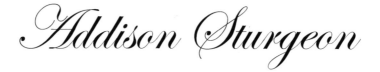

CHAPTER 3: OVERCOMING COMMON CHALLENGES

Embarking on a journey with intermittent fasting, especially for women over 50, is not without its hurdles. As we delve into this lifestyle, we encounter common challenges that can seem daunting at first. Hunger pangs, social eating scenarios, and adjusting to a new eating schedule are just a few of the obstacles that might arise. Yet, these challenges do not need to be roadblocks. Instead, they can become stepping stones to mastering this health-enhancing practice.

In this chapter, we explore the typical challenges faced when adopting intermittent fasting and offer practical solutions to navigate these waters smoothly. Like any significant lifestyle change, intermittent fasting requires adaptation and patience. It's about learning how to listen to your body, understanding your limits, and finding ways to integrate fasting into your life that feel both natural and sustainable.

We'll share insights on how to effectively manage hunger without compromising your goals, how to partake in family meals and social gatherings without feeling isolated or restricted, and how to adjust your fasting plan to accommodate health conditions that may require special consideration.

Remember, the path to wellness through intermittent fasting isn't about perfection. It's about progression. It's about building resilience and flexibility in your approach to health. As we tackle each of these common challenges, you'll find that with each small victory, you're not just overcoming a temporary obstacle; you're laying the foundation for a healthier, more vibrant future. This chapter is dedicated to helping you turn potential setbacks into opportunities for growth and empowerment, ensuring that your fasting journey is as rewarding as it is healthful.

3.1 DEALING WITH HUNGER AND CRAVINGS

For many embarking on the intermittent fasting journey, dealing with hunger and cravings represents a formidable challenge. These sensations, though natural, often become heightened obstacles when you're adjusting to a new eating schedule. Understanding the physiological and psychological factors that drive hunger and cravings can equip you with the tools to manage them effectively and maintain your fasting regimen without feeling overwhelmed.

Understanding Hunger and Cravings

Hunger is a physiological need signaling that your body requires nutrients, while cravings are often psychological, arising from habits, environmental triggers, or emotional states. During intermittent fasting, you might experience both as your body adjusts to new meal times and reduced caloric intake. It's important to discern between the two because they require different strategies to manage.

Strategies to Manage Hunger

1. Gradual Transition into Fasting: Jumping straight into a strict fasting regimen can shock your body and increase hunger pangs. Instead, ease into fasting gradually. If you're planning to adopt the 16/8 method, start by delaying breakfast for an hour and gradually increase the delay over several days until you reach your desired fasting window.

2. Optimal Nutrient Intake: During your eating window, focus on meals rich in fiber, protein, and healthy fats. These macronutrients are not only satiating but also take longer to digest, which helps sustain your energy levels and fullness for extended periods. For instance, incorporating foods like avocados, legumes, whole grains, lean proteins, and nuts can significantly reduce feelings of hunger during your fasting periods.

3. Stay Hydrated: Often, feelings of hunger are actually signs of dehydration. Ensure you drink adequate amounts of water throughout the day. Herbal teas and black coffee are also excellent for keeping hunger at bay during fasting periods, as they can help fill the void without adding calories.

Managing Cravings

1. Identify Triggers: Cravings are frequently triggered by specific emotional or environmental cues. Identifying these triggers can be a powerful step in managing your response to them. For example, if you find you crave sweets mid-afternoon, it could be due to a drop in blood sugar levels, boredom, or habit.

2. Healthy Substitutions: When cravings hit, having healthy alternatives is key. Instead of reaching for sugary snacks, opt for fresh fruits, nuts, or yogurt. These not only satisfy your cravings but also provide valuable nutrients that support your overall health.

3. Mindful Eating: Practice being present while eating. Mindful eating helps you enjoy your food more and increases your awareness of fullness cues, which can help prevent overeating and indulging in cravings mindlessly.

Psychological Strategies

1. Cognitive Reframing: Change the way you think about fasting and hunger. Rather than seeing fasting as a denial of food, view it as a positive lifestyle choice that contributes to your longevity and well-being. This mindset shift can make the experience feel empowering rather than punitive.

2. Stress Management: Since emotional distress can exacerbate hunger and cravings, incorporating stress-reduction techniques such as meditation, yoga, or deep-breathing exercises can be very beneficial.

3. Support System: Embarking on an intermittent fasting journey can be challenging, so it's helpful to have a support system. Sharing your experiences with friends who are also fasting or joining online support groups can provide motivation and practical tips for coping with hunger and cravings.

Long-term Adaptation

Over time, as your body adapts to the fasting schedule, you will notice a natural decrease in hunger and cravings. This adaptation phase varies by individual but typically settles down as your body becomes accustomed to new eating patterns and as you implement the strategies outlined.

Intermittent fasting isn't just about enduring hunger and suppressing cravings—it's about learning to listen to and understand your body's signals, nourishing it appropriately, and finding a rhythm that aligns with your life. By addressing both the physiological and psychological aspects of hunger and cravings, you can make intermittent fasting a sustainable and beneficial part of your lifestyle, turning what seems like a challenge into an opportunity for growth and health optimization.

3.2 MANAGING SOCIAL AND FAMILY MEALS

Navigating social and family meals while maintaining an intermittent fasting schedule can feel like walking a tightrope. It's about balancing personal health commitments with the joy of sharing meals and making memories with loved ones. This subchapter is dedicated to strategies that allow you to honor your fasting regimen without missing out on these valuable moments.

Understanding the Social Dynamics

Food is more than sustenance; it's a cornerstone of social interaction and familial bonding. Dinners, brunches, and holiday meals are often laden with expectations and traditions that can pose challenges for those practicing intermittent fasting. The key to managing these situations is preparation and flexibility.

Flexibility is Key

One of the most effective strategies is to plan your fasting windows around anticipated social events. If you know you have a family dinner, consider adjusting your eating window to accommodate this. This might mean shifting your fasting period earlier in the day or delaying it until after the meal. The flexibility of intermittent fasting is one of its greatest strengths—you can tailor it to fit your life, not the other way around.

Communicating Your Needs

Open communication with family and friends about your fasting schedule can mitigate awkwardness and build support. Explain why you are fasting and the health benefits you hope to achieve. Most people will understand and respect your decisions if they are framed in terms of personal health and well-being. It's also helpful to emphasize that this diet change is not a judgment of their eating habits or traditions but a personal choice for your health.

Choosing Your Battles

Not every meal needs to be a battleground for sticking strictly to your fasting schedule. Sometimes, it's okay to make exceptions. If it's a special occasion like a birthday or anniversary, you might decide to participate fully and return to your regular fasting routine the next day. This approach can relieve psychological stress and improve adherence to intermittent fasting in the long run.

Bringing Your Own Food

In situations where adjusting your fasting schedule isn't feasible, consider bringing your own food that fits within your dietary requirements. This can be especially useful for potluck-style gatherings. Contributing a dish that you can eat allows you to participate without breaking your fast early.

Mindful Eating During Social Meals

When you do choose to eat in a social setting, practice mindful eating. Focus on enjoying the quality of the food rather than the quantity. Savor each bite and listen to your body's cues about fullness and satisfaction. This practice not only enhances your dining experience but also helps prevent overeating, which is common in social settings.

Dealing with Peer Pressure

Sometimes, the biggest challenge is resisting the well-meaning but persistent offers of food from others. Prepare a few polite but firm responses to decline offers that don't fit your fasting schedule or dietary choices. Phrases like "I'm really focusing on my health right now" or "I've already eaten, but everything looks wonderful!" can be helpful.

Incorporating Buffer Strategies

Another tactic is to include buffer strategies such as starting with a salad or a broth-based soup if you find yourself needing to break your fast earlier than planned. These foods are filling but low in calories, helping you ease into the meal without consuming too much too quickly.

Staying Positive and Encouraging

Maintaining a positive attitude about your fasting lifestyle can encourage others to be supportive. Share your successes and how you feel healthier, which can turn curiosity into cheerleading from your social circle.

Long-Term Sustainability

Ultimately, the goal is to integrate intermittent fasting into your life in a way that feels sustainable and positive. This means finding ways to navigate social meals without feeling socially isolated or nutritionally compromised. With careful planning, open communication, and a flexible approach, it is entirely possible to enjoy the rich social tapestry of shared meals while adhering to your fasting plan.

Conclusion

Balancing intermittent fasting with social and family meals doesn't have to be a source of stress. By planning ahead, communicating openly, and applying flexible strategies, you can enjoy the best of both worlds—maintaining your health commitments while fully engaging in joyful social interactions. This approach not only enhances your ability to stick with intermittent fasting but also enriches your social life, proving that health and happiness can indeed go hand in hand.

3.3 ADJUSTING YOUR FASTING PLAN FOR HEALTH ISSUES

Embracing intermittent fasting is akin to embarking on a personalized health journey—one that must adapt to the ever-changing landscape of your body's needs, particularly when faced with health issues. Whether managing a chronic condition or navigating the fluctuations of an acute illness, the adaptability of your fasting regimen can play a crucial role in maintaining overall health while ensuring your body receives the care it requires.

Recognizing Individual Health Needs

Health is a dynamic state, influenced by various factors including age, genetic predisposition, lifestyle choices, and pre-existing medical conditions. When adopting or maintaining an intermittent fasting schedule, it's crucial to consider these elements as they significantly impact how your body responds to fasting.

Consulting Healthcare Professionals

Before making any significant changes to your fasting regimen, especially when dealing with health issues, the first step should always be to consult with a healthcare provider. Doctors, dietitians, and other health specialists can offer invaluable advice tailored to your specific health status and needs. They can help determine whether intermittent fasting is advisable and guide how to adjust it to complement any treatments or medications you may be on.

Flexible Fasting Plans

Flexibility is essential when adjusting your fasting plan to accommodate health issues. For some, traditional fasting windows like the 16/8 method may become impractical or uncomfortable. In such cases, shorter fasting periods or less frequent fasting days might be more appropriate. Listening to your body and being willing to modify your approach is key to integrating fasting into your life as health circumstances change.

Managing Chronic Conditions

For those with chronic conditions such as diabetes, heart disease, or autoimmune disorders, intermittent fasting requires careful management. Balancing nutrient intake during eating windows becomes crucial to avoid exacerbating these conditions. For instance, people with diabetes need to manage their blood sugar levels carefully to prevent both hyperglycemia and hypoglycemia, which might involve adjusting the timing and composition of meals around their fasting periods.

Addressing Medication Schedules

Medication regimes often need to be closely coordinated with meal timings, especially for medications that require intake with food or have specific nutritional interactions. Adjusting fasting windows to align with medication schedules is important to maintain the effectiveness of your medication while practicing intermittent fasting. This might mean having a larger eating window or timing your medication to coincide with meals during your eating periods.

Handling Acute Illnesses

During acute illnesses, such as infections or temporary medical conditions, the body requires more energy and often more nutrients to facilitate recovery. It's generally advisable to pause intermittent fasting during such times to allow your body to focus on healing. Once you have recovered, you can gradually reintroduce fasting into your routine, ideally under medical guidance.

Psychological and Physical Monitoring

Regular monitoring of both physical and psychological health is crucial when adjusting your fasting plan for health issues. Physical symptoms like fatigue, dizziness, or abnormal weight loss can indicate that adjustments are necessary. Similarly, psychological effects such as increased stress or anxiety about eating and fasting schedules should not be overlooked. Maintaining a diary or log where you can note these symptoms along with your fasting schedule can be helpful in tracking patterns that necessitate adjustments.

Nutritional Adequacy

Ensuring nutritional adequacy is paramount, especially when health issues are present. Each meal during your eating window should be rich in essential nutrients to support overall health and address specific dietary needs related to your condition. Consulting with a dietitian can help in planning meals that maximize nutrient intake while adhering to your fasting schedule.

Gradual Resumption After Health Setbacks

If you need to pause your fasting practice due to health concerns, the resumption should be as gradual as the initial adaptation phase. This cautious approach helps prevent undue strain on your body and allows you to gauge how your health responds to reintroduced fasting.

Adjusting your intermittent fasting plan in response to health issues is a thoughtful process that requires awareness, flexibility, and professional guidance. It's about finding a balance that maintains the integrity of your fasting regimen while accommodating the unique health challenges you face. With the right adjustments, intermittent fasting can continue to be a beneficial part of your health management strategy, supporting both your physical and mental well-being through various stages of health and life.

CHAPTER 4: NUTRITION AND SUPPLEMENT GUIDE

As we embrace the practice of intermittent fasting, understanding the synergy between nutrition and fasting cycles becomes paramount. This chapter delves into the essential world of nutrition and supplements, guiding you on how to nourish your body effectively during your eating windows to maximize the health benefits of your fasting regimen.

Nutrition isn't just about eating; it's about feeding your body the right way, especially during the times you do eat. For women over 50, this becomes even more crucial, as the body's needs for certain nutrients increase, while the efficiency of absorbing these nutrients may decrease. This guide is designed to equip you with the knowledge to choose foods and supplements that not only fill you up but also fulfill your body's varied nutritional needs.

Here, we'll explore how to ensure that each meal provides the vitamins, minerals, proteins, and other nutrients necessary to support your health. We'll break down the roles of key nutrients, identify which ones you need more of, and discuss how to get them. This includes a look at dietary sources, as well as when and why you might consider supplements.

Moreover, the guide will address common nutritional challenges that arise with age, such as changes in digestive efficiency and bone density, and how intermittent fasting can be tailored to help mitigate these issues. We'll also cover the importance of hydration and electrolyte balance, which are crucial for maintaining energy levels and overall health during fasting periods.

The goal is to make your eating periods as impactful as possible, turning each meal into an opportunity for nourishing and revitalizing your body. This isn't just about maintaining health as you age—it's about enhancing it, giving you the vitality and energy to enjoy every moment of your later years.

4.1 ESSENTIAL NUTRIENTS AND SUPPLEMENTS FOR WOMEN OVER 50

As women transition into their fifties and beyond, their nutritional needs evolve, necessitating a focused approach to diet that not only prevents nutrient deficiencies but also supports overall health, vitality, and longevity. Understanding the essential nutrients and when to supplement is pivotal in creating a nutritional plan that complements the benefits of intermittent fasting. This comprehensive guide aims to illuminate the key nutrients and supplements that are particularly beneficial for women over 50.

Understanding Nutritional Needs

The nutritional landscape for women over 50 changes due to a variety of physiological shifts. Decreased bone density, changes in blood pressure, and altered metabolic rates are just a few of the issues that can be mitigated through a targeted nutritional strategy. The focus here is not just on avoiding deficiency but on optimizing health.

Calcium and Vitamin D

Calcium and vitamin D top the list of essential nutrients for women over 50, primarily due to their role in bone health. As estrogen levels decline with age, bone density decreases, increasing the risk of osteoporosis. Calcium supports bone structure, while vitamin D enhances calcium absorption. Ideally, calcium intake should come from dietary sources like dairy products, leafy greens, and fortified foods. However, if dietary intake falls short, supplements might be necessary, especially for vitamin D, which many individuals are deficient in due to limited sun exposure.

Magnesium

Magnesium is another crucial mineral, particularly for aging women. It supports muscle and nerve function, helps regulate blood pressure, and is vital for the metabolic process. Magnesium also plays a role in converting the food we eat into energy and creating new proteins from amino acids. It is found in foods like nuts, seeds, whole grains, and leafy green vegetables. Considering its critical functions and the commonality of magnesium deficiency, supplementing this nutrient can be beneficial if dietary intake is insufficient.

Omega-3 Fatty Acids

Omega-3 fatty acids are essential fats that the body cannot produce on its own. They are crucial for maintaining heart health, reducing inflammation, and supporting brain health. As cognitive decline is a concern for the aging population, omega-3s are especially important. While fatty fish like salmon and sardines are the best sources, fish oil supplements can be an effective alternative for those who don't consume enough through their diet.

B Vitamins

The B vitamins, including B12, folate, and B6, play integral roles in overall energy levels, brain function, and cell metabolism. Vitamin B12, in particular, is vital for creating red blood cells and DNA, and its absorption decreases with age due to changes in stomach acid production. Foods rich in B12 include meat, fish, and dairy products. For vegetarians or those with decreased absorption, B12 supplements are often recommended.

Fiber

Fiber isn't just crucial for digestive health; it also plays a role in regulating blood sugar levels and lowering cholesterol. As metabolism slows with age, maintaining a diet high in fiber can help manage weight and reduce the risk of developing type 2 diabetes. Foods rich in fiber include whole grains, vegetables, fruits, and legumes. For those struggling to meet their fiber needs through diet alone, a fiber supplement might be an appropriate addition.

Antioxidants: Vitamin C and E

Antioxidants such as vitamins C and E help combat oxidative stress and inflammation, factors that contribute to aging and chronic diseases. Vitamin C is pivotal for skin health and immune function, while vitamin E supports eye health and skin repair. Both can be sourced from a variety of fruits and vegetables like oranges, strawberries, almonds, and sunflower seeds. Supplementing with these vitamins can be beneficial when dietary intake is lacking, especially in the case of vitamin E, which is less abundant in foods.

Probiotics

Probiotics are beneficial bacteria that promote digestive health and support the immune system. As gut health often declines with age, incorporating probiotics can be beneficial. They are found in fermented foods like yogurt, kefir, and sauerkraut. For those who do not consume these foods regularly, probiotic supplements can be a valuable addition to maintain gut flora balance.

Creating a Balanced Approach

Incorporating these nutrients into your diet requires a balanced approach that considers your overall health, dietary preferences, and any specific medical considerations. It's essential to tailor your nutrient intake to support your body's changing needs, enhancing the effects of intermittent fasting and promoting a vibrant, healthful lifestyle.

In conclusion, for women over 50, paying close attention to these essential nutrients and understanding when supplementation is beneficial can significantly enhance the quality of life and support healthy aging. Whether through diet or supplements, the goal is to provide the body with the best resources to thrive during fasting and feeding alike.

4.2 HYDRATION AND ELECTROLYTE BALANCE DURING FASTING

In the realm of intermittent fasting, maintaining hydration and proper electrolyte balance is not just a health requirement; it is an art that enhances the fasting experience, aiding in everything from detoxification to energy levels and cognitive function. For women over 50, who may already face challenges like hormonal changes and increased risk of osteoporosis, hydration and electrolyte management take on added importance.

Understanding Hydration and Electrolyte Balance

Hydration during intermittent fasting is crucial because water serves multiple roles in the body, including regulating body temperature, helping with metabolic processes, and assisting in detoxification. Water is the transporter of nutrients and waste in and out of cells, making it essential for maintaining health during the metabolic switch that occurs during fasting periods.

Electrolytes, including sodium, potassium, calcium, and magnesium, are charged minerals that help maintain the body's fluid balance, nerve transmission, and muscle function. When you fast, your body's electrolyte balance can be disrupted, particularly as insulin levels drop and the body begins to shed excess sodium and water.

The Hydration Strategy During Fasting

The key to effective hydration during fasting is not merely to drink when you feel thirsty but to maintain a consistent intake throughout the day. Aim for around 8-10 cups of fluids daily, which can come from water, herbal teas, and other non-caloric beverages. It's important to start your day with a good hydration base, especially if your eating window is later in the day.

Recognizing Dehydration Signs

Understanding the signs of dehydration can help you manage your hydration more effectively. Common symptoms include headaches, dry mouth, dizziness, and darker urine. During fasting, you might overlook these signs, mistaking them for normal fasting side effects, but addressing them quickly by increasing fluid intake is essential.

Electrolytes and Fasting

Electrolyte balance can be particularly challenging during longer fasting periods as the body adjusts its mineral needs. Drinking electrolyte-infused waters or incorporating a pinch of Himalayan pink salt in your water can help maintain sodium levels, which is vital since sodium is often flushed out when insulin levels drop during fasting.

Potassium is another critical electrolyte, involved in muscle functions and heart health. Low potassium levels can lead to fatigue, muscle cramps, and heart palpitations. Foods rich in potassium, such as avocados, spinach, and mushrooms, should be included during your eating windows. In some cases, supplementing with an electrolyte formula during fasting can be beneficial, especially for longer fasts.

The Role of Magnesium and Calcium

Magnesium supports over 300 enzymatic reactions in the body and helps with energy production, which can be particularly beneficial during fasting. It also aids in the management of potassium and calcium within the body, making it a critical electrolyte for overall balance. Including magnesium-rich foods like nuts, seeds, and whole grains in your diet can help, and magnesium supplements can be considered based on dietary intake and medical advice.

Calcium's role extends beyond bone health; it is crucial for proper muscle function and nerve transmission. Ensuring adequate calcium intake during eating periods is vital, especially to combat the accelerated bone density loss seen in postmenopausal women.

Practical Tips for Hydration and Electrolyte Balance

1. **Begin Your Day with Water**: Starting with a large glass of water can jump-start hydration and help mitigate any overnight fluid deficits.
2. **Flavor Your Water**: Adding slices of cucumber, lemon, or mint can make drinking water more enjoyable, encouraging you to consume more throughout the day.
3. **Monitor Your Intake**: Keep track of your fluid intake to ensure you're meeting your daily hydration goals, especially on hot days or when exercising.
4. **Adjust According to Your Body's Signals**: Be responsive to your body's needs. If you feel symptoms of electrolyte imbalance, consider adjusting your intake of electrolyte-rich foods or supplements.
5. **Consult with a Healthcare Provider**: Before adding any supplements to your diet, especially if you have health conditions like kidney disease or cardiovascular issues, consult with a healthcare professional.

Proper hydration and electrolyte management form the cornerstone of a successful fasting experience. By ensuring these elements are in balance, you empower your body to handle the physiological demands of intermittent fasting, supporting your overall health goals and enhancing the efficacy of your fasting regimen.

4.3 PREBIOTICS AND PROBIOTICS FOR GUT HEALTH

The gut is often referred to as the "second brain" of the body, indicative of its crucial role not just in digestion but in overall health and well-being. For women over 50, maintaining a healthy gut becomes increasingly important as changes in metabolism and immune function become more pronounced. This is where prebiotics and probiotics step into the spotlight, offering a pathway to enhanced digestive health and beyond.

Understanding Prebiotics and Probiotics

Prebiotics are non-digestible fibers that serve as fuel for probiotics—the beneficial bacteria residing in your gut. They help probiotics thrive and multiply, enhancing the gut microbiome's overall health and functionality. Probiotics, on the other hand, are live bacteria found in certain foods and supplements that can provide numerous health benefits when consumed in adequate amounts.

The Role of Prebiotics

Prebiotics are found naturally in many foods, including bananas, onions, garlic, leeks, asparagus, artichokes, and whole grains. Incorporating these foods into your diet can help foster a healthy environment for beneficial gut bacteria to grow. This is particularly important during intermittent fasting, as the timing of food intake can influence the gut flora's balance.

The benefits of prebiotics extend beyond simple digestion. They have been shown to improve mineral absorption, enhance the immune system, and could even help regulate mood and reduce stress—a factor that can significantly impact gut health.

The Benefits of Probiotics

Probiotics have been celebrated for their ability to restore and maintain the health of the gut microbiome. This is crucial for preventing and managing conditions common in women over 50, such as irritable bowel syndrome (IBS) and chronic constipation. Probiotics are particularly beneficial in maintaining a healthy digestive system, which can be affected by the hormonal changes and slowed metabolism that accompany menopause.

The strains Lactobacillus and Bifidobacterium are particularly beneficial for digestive health. These can be found in fermented foods like yogurt, kefir, sauerkraut, and kombucha, which can easily be incorporated into your eating periods when practicing intermittent fasting.

Probiotics and Immune Function

A robust immune system relies heavily on a healthy gut, as a significant portion of immune cells resides in the gut wall. Probiotics can enhance the gut's mucosal immune system, which protects against pathogens and maintains health. This is particularly important as the immune function tends to weaken with age, making older adults more susceptible to infections.

Managing Inflammation

Chronic inflammation is a root cause of many diseases associated with aging. Probiotics can play a role in managing and reducing systemic inflammation by enhancing the gut barrier, modulating the immune response, and reducing the presence of inflammation-inducing pathogens.

Incorporating Prebiotics and Probiotics into a Fasting Diet

Incorporating prebiotics and probiotics into your diet requires thoughtful planning, especially when you are intermittent fasting. It's important to include prebiotic-rich foods during your eating windows, ensuring that these fibers can aid probiotic bacteria in flourishing. For probiotics, dietary sources are generally recommended, but supplements can also be used, especially if dietary intake is not sufficient or if specific strains are needed.

Considerations for Supplementation

While dietary sources of prebiotics and probiotics are preferred, supplements can play a critical role in ensuring adequate intake. When choosing supplements, look for products containing live and active cultures, and consider factors such as the number of viable bacteria per dose and the inclusion of bacteria strains that are most beneficial for your health needs.

Monitoring Your Body's Response

As you integrate more prebiotic and probiotic foods into your diet, it's important to monitor how your body responds. Some people may experience gas, bloating, or discomfort, especially when increasing fiber intake rapidly. Adjusting the types and amounts of these foods gradually can help mitigate these effects.

For women over 50, prebiotics and probiotics offer a vital tool for maintaining gut health, enhancing immune function, and reducing the risk of chronic diseases. By understanding how to effectively incorporate these elements into your diet, particularly within the constraints and opportunities of intermittent fasting, you can significantly enhance not only your digestive health but your overall vitality and well-being. Through mindful inclusion of these powerful nutrients, you're not just feeding your gut—you're nourishing your entire body.

CHAPTER 5: BREAKFAST RECIPES

Breaking your fast each morning provides an exciting opportunity to nourish your body and set the tone for the day ahead. In this chapter, we explore breakfast recipes that are not only delicious and satisfying but are also tailored to align with the nutritional needs and fasting schedules of women over 50. Each recipe is crafted to maximize health benefits, emphasizing nutrients that support a vibrant, active lifestyle while considering the unique metabolic and dietary needs of aging gracefully.

Whether your fasting window ends in the early hours or closer to midday, the recipes featured here are designed to kickstart your metabolism, stabilize blood sugar, and provide sustained energy. They cater to a variety of tastes and preferences, ensuring that everyone can find something to enjoy. From nutrient-rich smoothies and shakes that can be prepared in minutes to high-protein dishes that rebuild and nourish, each recipe is a building block toward a healthier you.

Additionally, for those mornings when time is a luxury, quick and healthy options are available that don't compromise on nutritional value or taste. These meals are perfect for easing into your day without overwhelming preparation, making it possible to maintain your fasting routine without stress.

This collection of breakfast recipes aims to inspire and energize, proving that healthy eating can be simple, delicious, and perfectly suited to your intermittent fasting lifestyle. It's about more than just the first meal of the day—it's about crafting a morning ritual that you look forward to, one that fuels both your body and your spirit for whatever the day holds.

5.1 NUTRIENT-RICH SMOOTHIES AND SHAKES

Smoothies and shakes are wonderful options for breaking your fast, providing a refreshing, nutrient-packed start to your day that's easy to prepare and digest. These recipes are designed to include a blend of proteins, healthy fats, and fibers along with vitamins and minerals tailored to support the metabolism and energy levels of women over 50. Each smoothie or shake is crafted to deliver maximum nutrition while being easy on the digestive system, making them perfect for the first meal of the day in an intermittent fasting routine.

ANTIOXIDANT BERRY FLAX SMOOTHIE

PREPARATION TIME: 5 min - **COOKING TIME:** 0 min **MODE OF COOKING:** Blending - **SERVINGS:** 1 **INGREDIENTS:**
- 1 cup mixed berries (blueberries, strawberries, raspberries), fresh or frozen
- 1 Tbsp ground flaxseed
- 1 cup spinach leaves
- 1/2 banana
- 1 cup unsweetened almond milk
- 1 Tbsp almond butter

DIRECTIONS:
1. Combine all ingredients in a blender.
2. Blend on high until smooth.
3. Serve immediately.

TIPS:
- Use frozen berries to chill the smoothie without diluting it with ice.
- Adding almond butter provides a creamy texture and healthy fats.

N.V.: Calories: 295, Fat: 15g, Carbs: 35g, Protein: 8g, Sugar: 18g

GREEN DETOX SMOOTHIE

PREPARATION TIME: 5 min - **COOKING TIME:** 0 min **MODE OF COOKING:** Blending - **SERVINGS:** 1 **INGREDIENTS:**

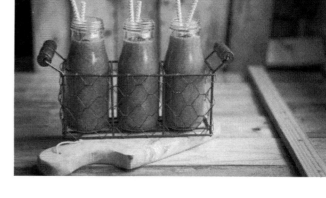

- 1 cup kale leaves, stems removed
- 1 small green apple, cored and sliced
- 1/2 cucumber, sliced
- Juice of 1/2 lemon
- 1 Tbsp chia seeds
- 1 cup coconut water

DIRECTIONS:
1. Place all ingredients in a blender.
2. Blend until smooth and creamy.
3. Serve chilled.

TIPS:
- Add a piece of ginger for extra zest and digestive benefits.
- Coconut water is hydrating and adds a natural sweetness.

N.V.: Calories: 180, Fat: 4g, Carbs: 33g, Protein: 4g, Sugar: 20g

PROTEIN POWER SHAKE

PREPARATION TIME: 5 min - **COOKING TIME:** 0 min **MODE OF COOKING:** Blending - **SERVINGS:** 1 **INGREDIENTS:**

- 1 scoop vanilla protein powder
- 1/2 avocado
- 1 cup unsweetened almond milk
- 1 tsp cinnamon
- 1 Tbsp flaxseeds
- Ice cubes (optional)

DIRECTIONS:
1. Place all ingredients in a blender.
2. Blend on high until smooth.
3. Serve immediately.

TIPS:
- Avocado adds creaminess and healthy fats, making this shake filling.
- Cinnamon can help regulate blood sugar levels.

N.V.: Calories: 300, Fat: 19g, Carbs: 21g, Protein: 21g, Sugar: 2g

TROPICAL TURMERIC SMOOTHIE

PREPARATION TIME: 5 min - **COOKING TIME:** 0 min **MODE OF COOKING:** Blending - **SERVINGS:** 1 **INGREDIENTS:**

- 1 cup pineapple chunks
- 1/2 mango, peeled and diced
- 1/2 tsp turmeric powder
- 1 Tbsp coconut oil
- 1 cup coconut milk

DIRECTIONS:
1. Combine all ingredients in a blender.
2. Blend until smooth.
3. Serve chilled.

TIPS:
- Turmeric adds anti-inflammatory properties and a vibrant color.
- Coconut oil provides healthy fats that boost metabolism.

N.V.: Calories: 310, Fat: 19g, Carbs: 35g, Protein: 3g, Sugar: 28g

MORNING MOCHA SHAKE

PREPARATION TIME: 5 min - **COOKING TIME:** 0 min **MODE OF COOKING:** Blending - **SERVINGS:** 1 **INGREDIENTS:**
- 1 cup brewed coffee, cooled
- 1/2 banana
- 1 Tbsp cocoa powder
- 1 Tbsp almond butter
- 1/2 cup Greek yogurt
- Ice cubes (optional)

DIRECTIONS:
1. Place all ingredients in a blender.
2. Blend on high until smooth.
3. Serve immediately.

TIPS:
- The banana adds natural sweetness and creaminess.
- Cocoa powder provides antioxidants without the added sugars of chocolate.

N.V.: Calories: 250, Fat: 12g, Carbs: 27g, Protein: 10g, Sugar: 15g

BLUEBERRY WALNUT BLISS SMOOTHIE

PREPARATION TIME: 5 min - **COOKING TIME:** 0 min **MODE OF COOKING:** Blending - **SERVINGS:** 1 **INGREDIENTS:**
- 1 cup blueberries, fresh or frozen
- 1/4 cup walnuts
- 1 cup spinach leaves
- 1/2 cup Greek yogurt
- 1 cup water

DIRECTIONS:
1. Combine all ingredients in a blender.
2. Blend until smooth.
3. Serve immediately.

TIPS:
- Walnuts add a boost of omega-3 fatty acids, which are great for heart health.
- Spinach is high in iron and blends well without overpowering the flavor.

N.V.: Calories: 295, Fat: 17g, Carbs: 27g, Protein: 12g, Sugar: 14g

These smoothies and shakes provide a delightful and nutritious way to break your fast, packed with ingredients designed to support your health and energy throughout the day.

AVOCADO LIME REFRESHER

PREPARATION TIME: 5 min - **COOKING TIME:** 0 min **MODE OF COOKING:** Blending - **SERVINGS:** 1 **INGREDIENTS:**
- 1 ripe avocado
- Juice of 1 lime
- 1 cup coconut water
- 1 handful of mint leaves

- 1 tbsp honey (optional)
- Ice cubes

DIRECTIONS:
1. Scoop the avocado flesh into a blender.
2. Add lime juice, coconut water, mint leaves, honey if using, and ice cubes.
3. Blend on high until smooth and frothy.
4. Serve chilled for a refreshing morning drink.

TIPS:
- Avocado provides a creamy texture and healthy fats that are excellent for heart health.
- Lime and mint offer a refreshing zest, perfect for waking up your senses in the morning.

N.V.: Calories: 240, Fat: 15g, Carbs: 27g, Protein: 3g, Sugar: 14g

SPICED PEAR GINGER SMOOTHIE

PREPARATION TIME: 5 min - **COOKING TIME:** 0 min **MODE OF COOKING:** Blending - **SERVINGS:** 1 **INGREDIENTS:**
- 1 ripe pear, cored and chopped
- 1/2 tsp freshly grated ginger
- 1/2 tsp cinnamon
- 1 cup almond milk
- 1 tbsp ground flaxseed
- Ice cubes

DIRECTIONS:
1. Combine pear, ginger, cinnamon, almond milk, and flaxseed in a blender.
2. Add ice cubes.
3. Blend until smooth and creamy.
4. Pour into a glass and enjoy a spiced, invigorating start to your day.

TIPS:
- Ginger adds a warming sensation, which can stimulate digestion and invigorate the senses.
- Cinnamon helps to regulate blood sugar levels, making this smoothie ideal for sustained energy.

N.V.: Calories: 180, Fat: 4g, Carbs: 35g, Protein: 2g, Sugar: 20g

CHOCOLATE BANANA PROTEIN SHAKE

PREPARATION TIME: 5 min - **COOKING TIME:** 0 min **MODE OF COOKING:** Blending - **SERVINGS:** 1 **INGREDIENTS:**
- 1 ripe banana
- 1 tbsp cocoa powder
- 1 scoop chocolate protein powder
- 1 cup oat milk
- Ice cubes

DIRECTIONS:
1. Place banana, cocoa powder, protein powder, and oat milk in a blender.
2. Add ice cubes.
3. Blend until smooth.
4. Serve immediately for a decadent but healthy start to your day.

TIPS:
- Choose a protein powder that complements your dietary preferences, such as whey or pea protein.
- Oat milk adds a mild sweetness and contributes additional fiber.

N.V.: Calories: 325, Fat: 4g, Carbs: 55g, Protein: 20g, Sugar: 25g

5.2 HIGH-PROTEIN BREAKFAST IDEAS

High-protein breakfasts are essential for women over 50, helping to maintain muscle mass, support bone health, and regulate blood sugar levels throughout the day. This selection of high-protein breakfast ideas is designed to provide a satisfying start to your day, combining both flavor and nutrition. Each recipe focuses on protein-rich ingredients, from eggs and dairy to nuts and seeds, ensuring you receive a balanced intake that supports your energy levels and nutritional needs during intermittent fasting.

SAVORY MUSHROOM AND SPINACH OMELETTE

PREPARATION TIME: 10 min - **COOKING TIME:** 10 min **MODE OF COOKING:** Sautéing - **SERVINGS:** 1 **INGREDIENTS:**

- 3 large eggs
- 1 cup fresh spinach, chopped
- 1/2 cup mushrooms, sliced
- 1/4 cup feta cheese, crumbled
- 1 Tbsp olive oil
- Salt and pepper to taste

DIRECTIONS:

1. Heat olive oil in a skillet over medium heat.
2. Sauté mushrooms until they are soft, about 5 minutes.
3. Add spinach and cook until wilted.
4. Beat the eggs with salt and pepper, and pour over the vegetables in the skillet.
5. Sprinkle feta cheese on top and let the eggs set around the edges before folding the omelette.
6. Serve hot.

TIPS:

- Cooking the vegetables before adding the eggs brings out their flavor and ensures they are fully cooked.
- Use a well-oiled or non-stick pan to prevent sticking.

N.V.: Calories: 400, Fat: 29g, Carbs: 6g, Protein: 28g, Sugar: 3g

COTTAGE CHEESE AND CHIVE PANCAKES

PREPARATION TIME: 15 min - **COOKING TIME:** 15 min **MODE OF COOKING:** Pan-frying - **SERVINGS:** 2 **INGREDIENTS:**

- 1 cup cottage cheese
- 2 large eggs
- 1/2 cup whole wheat flour
- 1/4 cup milk
- 2 Tbsp chives, finely chopped
- 1/2 tsp baking powder
- Salt to taste
- Butter, for cooking

DIRECTIONS:

1. In a bowl, mix cottage cheese, eggs, and milk until well combined.
2. Add flour, baking powder, chives, and salt to the cottage cheese mixture and stir until just combined.
3. Heat a non-stick skillet over medium heat and melt a small amount of butter.
4. Pour 1/4 cup of batter for each pancake and cook until bubbles form on the surface, then flip and cook until golden brown.
5. Serve warm with a dollop of sour cream or Greek yogurt.

TIPS:

- Do not overmix the batter to keep the pancakes fluffy.
- Serve with smoked salmon on top for an extra boost of protein.

N.V.: Calories: 315, Fat: 12g, Carbs: 25g, Protein: 23g, Sugar: 5g

SMOKED SALMON AND AVOCADO TOAST

PREPARATION TIME: 5 min - **COOKING TIME:** 0 min **MODE OF COOKING:** Assembling - **SERVINGS:** 1 **INGREDIENTS:**

- 2 slices whole-grain bread, toasted
- 4 oz smoked salmon
- 1 ripe avocado, sliced
- 1 Tbsp cream cheese
- 1 tsp lemon juice
- Fresh dill, for garnish
- Salt and black pepper to taste

DIRECTIONS:

1. Spread each slice of toasted bread with cream cheese.
2. Top with sliced avocado and smoked salmon.
3. Sprinkle lemon juice, salt, and black pepper over the top.
4. Garnish with fresh dill and serve immediately.

TIPS:

- Opt for high-quality smoked salmon for the best flavor and texture.
- Drizzle with a bit of extra virgin olive oil for added richness.

N.V.: Calories: 480, Fat: 29g, Carbs: 32g, Protein: 27g, Sugar: 5g

GREEK YOGURT PARFAIT WITH MIXED NUTS AND BERRIES

PREPARATION TIME: 5 min - **COOKING TIME:** 0 min **MODE OF COOKING:** Assembling - **SERVINGS:** 1 **INGREDIENTS:**

- 1 cup Greek yogurt
- 1/4 cup mixed berries (blueberries, raspberries, strawberries)
- 1/4 cup mixed nuts (almonds, walnuts, pecans), chopped
- 1 Tbsp honey
- 1/4 tsp cinnamon

DIRECTIONS:

1. In a serving bowl, layer half the Greek yogurt.
2. Add a layer of mixed berries and nuts.
3. Repeat with the remaining yogurt, berries, and nuts.
4. Drizzle honey over the top and sprinkle with cinnamon.
5. Serve immediately or refrigerate until ready to eat.

TIPS:

- For added texture, you can include a layer of granola.
- Adjust the sweetness by increasing or decreasing the amount of honey based on preference.

N.V.: Calories: 420, Fat: 20g, Carbs: 36g, Protein: 24g, Sugar: 18g

SPINACH AND FETA BREAKFAST WRAP

PREPARATION TIME: 10 min - **COOKING TIME:** 5 min **MODE OF COOKING:** Sautéing and wrapping - **SERVINGS:** 1 **INGREDIENTS:**

- 2 eggs, beaten
- 1 cup fresh spinach
- 1/4 cup feta cheese, crumbled
- 1 whole wheat tortilla
- 1 Tbsp olive oil
- Salt and pepper to taste

DIRECTIONS:

1. Heat olive oil in a skillet over medium heat.
2. Add spinach and sauté until wilted, about 2 minutes.
3. Pour beaten eggs over spinach, season with salt and pepper, and stir gently until the eggs are set.
4. Sprinkle feta cheese over the eggs and remove from heat.
5. Place the egg mixture on the tortilla, roll it up, and serve.

TIPS:

- Wrap can be made ahead and reheated for a quick and nutritious breakfast.
- Add diced tomatoes or onions for extra flavor and nutrients.

N.V.: Calories: 410, Fat: 27g, Carbs: 24g, Protein: 22g, Sugar: 3g

TURKEY AND EGG BREAKFAST BURRITO

PREPARATION TIME: 10 min - **COOKING TIME:** 10 min **MODE OF COOKING:** Sautéing and wrapping - **SERVINGS:** 1 **INGREDIENTS:**

- 1 whole wheat tortilla
- 2 eggs, beaten
- 2 oz lean turkey breast, cooked and chopped
- 1/4 cup black beans, rinsed and drained
- 2 Tbsp cheddar cheese, shredded
- 1/4 avocado, sliced
- 1 Tbsp salsa
- Salt and pepper to taste
- 1 tsp olive oil

DIRECTIONS:

1. Heat olive oil in a non-stick skillet over medium heat.
2. Add turkey and black beans to the skillet and cook until heated through, about 2-3 minutes.
3. Pour beaten eggs over the turkey and beans, season with salt and pepper, and scramble until the eggs are cooked.
4. Warm the tortilla in a separate pan or in the microwave.
5. Place the egg mixture in the center of the tortilla, top with cheese, avocado slices, and salsa.
6. Fold the tortilla to enclose the filling and serve.

TIPS:

- Customize the burrito with additional vegetables like bell peppers or onions for added flavor.
- For a lower calorie option, use egg whites instead of whole eggs.

N.V.: Calories: 500, Fat: 26g, Carbs: 38g, Protein: 33g, Sugar: 4g

QUINOA AND EGG POWER BOWL

PREPARATION TIME: 5 min - **COOKING TIME:** 20 min **MODE OF COOKING:** Boiling and sautéing - **SERVINGS:** 1 **INGREDIENTS:**

- 1/2 cup quinoa
- 1 cup water
- 2 large eggs
- 1 cup spinach leaves
- 1/4 cup cherry tomatoes, halved
- 1 Tbsp olive oil
- Salt and pepper to taste
- 1 Tbsp pumpkin seeds

DIRECTIONS:

1. Rinse quinoa under cold water until water runs clear.

2. In a small pot, bring water to a boil. Add quinoa, reduce heat to low, cover, and simmer for 15 minutes until water is absorbed.
3. While quinoa cooks, heat olive oil in a skillet over medium heat. Sauté spinach until wilted, about 3-4 minutes.
4. In the same skillet, fry eggs to your preference.
5. Assemble the power bowl by placing cooked quinoa at the bottom. Top with sautéed spinach, cherry tomatoes, and fried eggs.
6. Season with salt and pepper and sprinkle pumpkin seeds over the top.

TIPS:
- Quinoa can be cooked in bulk and stored in the refrigerator for quick assembly of meals throughout the week.
- Add a drizzle of pesto or hot sauce for an extra flavor kick.

N.V.: Calories: 540, Fat: 30g, Carbs: 40g, Protein: 28g, Sugar: 3g

CHICKPEA AND AVOCADO TOAST

PREPARATION TIME: 10 min - **COOKING TIME:** 5 min **MODE OF COOKING:** Toasting and mashing - **SERVINGS:** 2 **INGREDIENTS:**
- 1 can (15 oz) chickpeas, drained and rinsed
- 1 ripe avocado
- Juice of 1 lemon
- 2 slices whole grain bread
- Salt and pepper to taste
- 1/2 tsp paprika
- Fresh parsley, chopped for garnish

DIRECTIONS:
1. In a bowl, mash the chickpeas and avocado together with lemon juice, salt, pepper, and paprika until well combined but still slightly chunky.
2. Toast the bread slices to your liking.
3. Spread the chickpea and avocado mixture evenly on each slice of toast.
4. Garnish with chopped parsley and serve immediately.

TIPS:
- For an extra protein boost, top with a poached or soft-boiled egg.
- This mixture can be made ahead and stored in the refrigerator for up to two days.

N.V.: Calories: 380, Fat: 20g, Carbs: 42g, Protein: 14g, Sugar: 6g

SWEET POTATO AND BLACK BEAN BREAKFAST BURRITOS

PREPARATION TIME: 15 min - **COOKING TIME:** 25 min **MODE OF COOKING:** Baking and wrapping - **SERVINGS:** 2 **INGREDIENTS:**
- 1 medium sweet potato, peeled and diced
- 1/2 cup black beans, cooked or canned
- 4 eggs, whisked
- 2 whole wheat tortillas
- 1/4 cup cheddar cheese, shredded
- 1/2 tsp cumin
- Salt and pepper to taste
- 1 Tbsp olive oil
- Salsa and sour cream, for serving

DIRECTIONS:
1. Preheat oven to 425°F (218°C). Toss diced sweet potatoes with olive oil, cumin, salt, and pepper. Spread on a baking sheet and bake for 20 minutes until tender.

2. In a skillet, scramble the eggs to your liking.
3. Warm tortillas in the microwave or on a skillet.
4. Assemble the burritos by dividing the roasted sweet potatoes, scrambled eggs, black beans, and cheddar cheese among the tortillas.
5. Roll up the tortillas, folding in the ends to enclose the filling.
6. Serve with salsa and sour cream on the side.

TIPS:
- Customize the burritos with additional vegetables like spinach or bell peppers for extra nutrients.
- These burritos can be wrapped in foil and stored in the fridge for a quick, reheat able breakfast option.

N.V.: Calories: 505, Fat: 25g, Carbs: 45g, Protein: 27g, Sugar: 8g

5.3 QUICK AND HEALTHY BREAKFAST BITES

In this section, we explore quick and healthy breakfast bites designed specifically for women over 50, who are balancing a busy lifestyle while maintaining a nutritious diet. Each recipe is crafted to be easy to prepare, ensuring that even on your busiest mornings, you can enjoy a breakfast that not only fuels your body efficiently but also aligns with your health goals. These bites are perfect for those who practice intermittent fasting or simply seek to enhance their morning routine with wholesome, energizing foods.

ALMOND BUTTER BANANA BITES

PREPARATION TIME: 5 min - **COOKING TIME:** 0 min **MODE OF COOKING:** Assembling - **SERVINGS: 2 INGREDIENTS:**
- 1 large banana
- 2 Tbsp almond butter
- 1/4 cup granola
- 1 Tbsp honey

DIRECTIONS:
1. Peel the banana and cut it into half-inch thick slices.
2. Spread almond butter on each banana slice.
3. Dip the almond butter side of each banana slice into granola.
4. Drizzle honey over the banana bites before serving.

TIPS:
- Choose a crunchy granola for added texture.
- For extra protein, sprinkle with chia seeds or crushed nuts.

N.V.: Calories: 210, Fat: 11g, Carbs: 27g, Protein: 4g, Sugar: 15g

GREEK YOGURT FRUIT CUPS

PREPARATION TIME: 10 min - **COOKING TIME:** 0 min **MODE OF COOKING:** Assembling - **SERVINGS: 4 INGREDIENTS:**
- 2 cups Greek yogurt
- 1/2 cup mixed berries (blueberries, strawberries, raspberries)
- 1/4 cup sliced almonds
- 2 Tbsp honey

DIRECTIONS:
1. Spoon Greek yogurt into four small cups.
2. Top each cup with an even distribution of mixed berries and sliced almonds.
3. Drizzle honey over each cup before serving.

TIPS:
- For a vegan option, use plant-based yogurt.
- Freeze for an hour before serving for a refreshing treat.

N.V.: Calories: 180, Fat: 9g, Carbs: 18g, Protein: 10g, Sugar: 14g

APPLE PEANUT BUTTER SANDWICHES

PREPARATION TIME: 5 min - **COOKING TIME:** 0 min **MODE OF COOKING:** Assembling - **SERVINGS:** 1 **INGREDIENTS:**

- 1 large apple, cored and sliced into rounds
- 2 Tbsp peanut butter
- 2 Tbsp granola
- 1 tsp honey (optional)

DIRECTIONS:

1. Spread peanut butter on one side of each apple slice.
2. Sprinkle granola over the peanut butter.
3. Top with another apple slice, peanut butter side facing down, to make a sandwich.
4. Drizzle with honey if desired.

TIPS:

- Choose a firm apple like Granny Smith or Fuji for best results.
- For added nutrition, include a sprinkle of flax seeds or hemp seeds in the granola.

N.V.: Calories: 325, Fat: 18g, Carbs: 36g, Protein: 8g, Sugar: 24g

SPINACH AND CHEESE EGG MUFFINS

PREPARATION TIME: 10 min - **COOKING TIME:** 20 min **MODE OF COOKING:** Baking - **SERVINGS:** 6 **INGREDIENTS:**

- 6 large eggs
- 1 cup fresh spinach, chopped
- 1/2 cup shredded cheddar cheese
- 1/4 cup milk
- Salt and pepper to taste
- Non-stick cooking spray

DIRECTIONS:

1. Preheat oven to 375°F (190°C).
2. Spray a muffin tin with non-stick cooking spray.
3. In a bowl, whisk together eggs, milk, salt, and pepper.
4. Stir in chopped spinach and shredded cheese.
5. Pour the egg mixture evenly into the muffin tin cavities.
6. Bake in the preheated oven for 20 minutes, or until the muffins are set and lightly golden on top.
7. Let cool slightly before removing from the tin.

TIPS:

- Add diced bell peppers or onions for extra flavor and nutrients.
- These muffins can be stored in the refrigerator for up to 4 days or frozen for longer storage.

N.V.: Calories: 150, Fat: 10g, Carbs: 2g, Protein: 12g, Sugar: 1g

OATMEAL AND CHIA SEED PUDDING

PREPARATION TIME: 5 min - **COOKING TIME:** 0 min (plus overnight refrigeration) **MODE OF COOKING:** Refrigerating - **SERVINGS:** 2 **INGREDIENTS:**

- 1 cup rolled oats
- 2 Tbsp chia seeds
- 2 cups almond milk
- 1 Tbsp maple syrup
- 1/2 tsp vanilla extract
- Fresh berries for topping

DIRECTIONS:

1. In a bowl, combine oats, chia seeds, almond milk, maple syrup, and vanilla extract.
2. Mix well until all ingredients are fully incorporated.
3. Cover and refrigerate overnight.
4. Before serving, stir the pudding, add more almond milk if needed, and top with fresh berries.

TIPS:

- Add a spoonful of nut butter for extra protein and flavor.
- Customize with different toppings like nuts, banana slices, or coconut flakes for variety.

N.V.: Calories: 280, Fat: 9g, Carbs: 44g, Protein: 8g, Sugar: 12g

COTTAGE CHEESE AND FRUIT PLATE

PREPARATION TIME: 5 min - **COOKING TIME:** 0 min **MODE OF COOKING:** Assembling - **SERVINGS:** 1 **INGREDIENTS:**

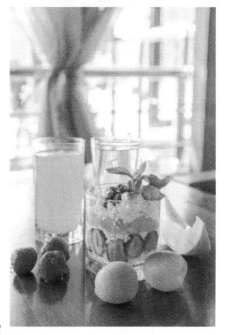

- 1 cup cottage cheese
- 1/2 cup sliced peaches
- 1/2 cup sliced strawberries
- 1 Tbsp honey
- 1 Tbsp sliced almonds

DIRECTIONS:

1. Place the cottage cheese in the center of a plate.
2. Arrange the sliced peaches and strawberries around the cottage cheese.
3. Drizzle honey over the fruit and cottage cheese.
4. Sprinkle sliced almonds on top.

TIPS:

- Opt for low-fat cottage cheese for a lighter option.
- Mix up the fruits seasonally for variety and freshness.

N.V.: Calories: 320, Fat: 8g, Carbs: 42g, Protein: 20g, Sugar: 32g

ZUCCHINI AND PARMESAN BREAKFAST PATTIES

PREPARATION TIME: 15 min - **COOKING TIME:** 10 min **MODE OF COOKING:** Pan-frying - **SERVINGS:** 4 **INGREDIENTS:**

- 2 cups grated zucchini (about 2 medium-sized zucchinis)
- 1/2 cup grated Parmesan cheese
- 1 large egg
- 1/4 cup whole wheat flour
- 1 garlic clove, minced
- Salt and pepper to taste
- 2 Tbsp olive oil for frying

DIRECTIONS:

1. Place the grated zucchini in a colander, sprinkle with salt, and let sit for 10 minutes. Squeeze out excess moisture.
2. In a bowl, combine the drained zucchini, Parmesan cheese, egg, flour, minced garlic, salt, and pepper. Mix until well combined.
3. Heat olive oil in a skillet over medium heat.
4. Form the zucchini mixture into small patties and fry for about 5 minutes on each side, until golden and crispy.
5. Drain on paper towels and serve warm.

TIPS:

- Serve these patties with a dollop of Greek yogurt or sour cream for added flavor.

- These patties can be made in advance and reheated for a quick breakfast.

N.V.: Calories: 180, Fat: 12g, Carbs: 10g, Protein: 8g, Sugar: 2g

ALMOND JOY OVERNIGHT OATS

PREPARATION TIME: 10 min - **COOKING TIME:** 0 min (plus overnight refrigeration) **MODE OF COOKING:** Refrigerating - **SERVINGS:** 2 **INGREDIENTS:**
- 1 cup rolled oats
- 1 cup coconut milk
- 1 Tbsp chia seeds
- 2 Tbsp shredded coconut
- 2 Tbsp slivered almonds
- 2 Tbsp dark chocolate chips
- 1 Tbsp honey or maple syrup

DIRECTIONS:
1. Combine rolled oats, coconut milk, chia seeds, shredded coconut, and honey in a mixing bowl.
2. Divide the mixture between two jars or containers.
3. Refrigerate overnight.
4. In the morning, top each serving with slivered almonds and dark chocolate chips before serving.

TIPS:
- For a lower sugar option, omit the chocolate chips and sweeten with a ripe banana mashed into the oat mixture before refrigerating.
- Stir well before eating to mix in all the flavors.

N.V.: Calories: 400, Fat: 22g, Carbs: 45g, Protein: 10g, Sugar: 18g

SUN-DRIED TOMATO AND SPINACH QUICHE CUPS

PREPARATION TIME: 15 min - **COOKING TIME:** 20 min **MODE OF COOKING:** Baking - **SERVINGS:** 6 **INGREDIENTS:**
- 6 large eggs
- 1/4 cup milk
- 1/2 cup sun-dried tomatoes, chopped
- 1 cup fresh spinach, chopped
- 1/4 cup feta cheese, crumbled
- Salt and pepper to taste
- Non-stick cooking spray

DIRECTIONS:
1. Preheat oven to 375°F (190°C). Spray a muffin tin with non-stick cooking spray.
2. In a large bowl, whisk together eggs and milk. Season with salt and pepper.
3. Stir in sun-dried tomatoes, spinach, and feta cheese.
4. Pour the mixture evenly into the prepared muffin tin.
5. Bake for 20 minutes, or until the eggs are set and the tops are slightly golden.
6. Let cool for a few minutes before removing from the tin.

TIPS:
- These quiche cups can be stored in the refrigerator for up to 4 days or frozen for longer storage.
- Reheat in the microwave for a quick and satisfying breakfast.

N.V.: Calories: 140, Fat: 9g, Carbs: 4g, Protein: 10g, Sugar: 2g

CHAPTER 6: LIGHT LUNCH RECIPES

In the journey toward vibrant health, particularly for women over 50, the role of a well-crafted lunch cannot be overstated. While breakfast may ignite the day's metabolic furnace, and dinner offers a reflective pause for nourishment, lunch serves as a critical bridge—fueling the body through the day's activities without weighing it down. In this chapter, we explore an array of light lunch recipes that harmonize beautifully with the body's midday needs, especially for those practicing intermittent fasting.

Each recipe is designed to be light yet satisfying, ensuring that you feel energized rather than sluggish as the day progresses. These meals integrate lean proteins, fiber-rich vegetables, and wholesome grains to provide balanced nutrition that supports metabolic health, bone density, and muscle maintenance—concerns that are particularly poignant for aging women.

From vibrant salads bursting with antioxidants to soothing soups and innovative wraps, these recipes are not only nourishing but also delight the palate and invigorate the spirit. They are quick to prepare, making them perfect for busy midday meals, whether you're at home or need to pack a lunch for outings or work. Each dish is also crafted to support dietary needs specific to women over 50, using ingredients that enhance energy levels, stabilize blood sugar, and provide vital nutrients to support overall health and well-being.

6.1 SALAD BOWLS FULL OF ANTIOXIDANTS

Salad bowls are not just about tossing greens on a plate; they are a canvas for creativity and a powerhouse of nutrients. This selection of salad bowls is designed specifically for women over 50, focusing on ingredients high in antioxidants, which play a crucial role in combating oxidative stress and enhancing overall health. Each recipe is packed with vibrant vegetables, lean proteins, and healthy fats to provide a balanced meal that supports energy levels and nourishes the body, while also being simple and quick to prepare for a rejuvenating lunch.

SUPER GREENS ANTIOXIDANT SALAD

PREPARATION TIME: 15 min - **COOKING TIME:** 0 min **MODE OF COOKING:** Assembling - **SERVINGS:** 2 **INGREDIENTS:**
- 2 cups mixed greens (spinach, kale, Swiss chard)
- 1/2 cup blueberries
- 1/4 cup walnuts, chopped
- 1/2 avocado, sliced
- 1/4 cup crumbled goat cheese
- 2 Tbsp flaxseeds
- 1/4 cup balsamic vinaigrette

DIRECTIONS:
1. In a large bowl, combine mixed greens, blueberries, and walnuts.
2. Top with avocado slices and crumbled goat cheese.
3. Sprinkle flaxseeds over the salad.
4. Drizzle balsamic vinaigrette evenly over the salad before serving.

TIPS:
- Massage kale leaves with a little olive oil to soften them if using raw.
- Toast walnuts for added flavor.

N.V.: Calories: 300, Fat: 25g, Carbs: 18g, Protein: 8g, Sugar: 7g

BEETROOT AND QUINOA ANTIOXIDANT BOWL

PREPARATION TIME: 10 min - **COOKING TIME:** 20 min **MODE OF COOKING:** Boiling - **SERVINGS:** 2 **INGREDIENTS:**

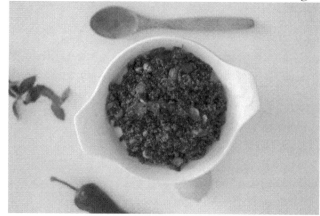

- 1 cup quinoa
- 2 cups water
- 1 medium beetroot, peeled and grated
- 1/2 cup carrot, grated
- 1/4 cup sunflower seeds
- 1/4 cup fresh parsley, chopped
- 2 Tbsp olive oil
- 1 lemon, juiced
- Salt and pepper to taste

DIRECTIONS:

1. Rinse quinoa under cold water until water runs clear.
2. In a pot, bring water to a boil. Add quinoa, reduce heat to low, cover, and cook for 15 minutes until fluffy.
3. In a large bowl, combine cooked quinoa, grated beetroot, and carrot.
4. Add sunflower seeds and chopped parsley.
5. Whisk together olive oil, lemon juice, salt, and pepper, and pour over the salad. Toss to coat evenly.
6. Serve chilled or at room temperature.

TIPS:

- Let the quinoa cool before adding to the salad to prevent wilting the greens.
- Squeeze a little extra lemon juice for added tanginess.

N.V.: Calories: 420, Fat: 22g, Carbs: 47g, Protein: 12g, Sugar: 6g

SPICY AVOCADO AND BLACK BEAN SALAD

PREPARATION TIME: 15 min - **COOKING TIME:** 0 min **MODE OF COOKING:** Assembling - **SERVINGS:** 2 **INGREDIENTS:**

- 1 can (15 oz) black beans, rinsed and drained
- 1 large avocado, diced
- 1/2 red bell pepper, diced
- 1/4 cup red onion, finely chopped
- 1 small jalapeño, seeded and minced
- 1/4 cup cilantro, chopped
- 2 Tbsp lime juice
- Salt and pepper to taste

DIRECTIONS:

1. In a large bowl, combine black beans, avocado, red bell pepper, red onion, and jalapeño.
2. Add chopped cilantro and drizzle with lime juice.
3. Season with salt and pepper and gently toss to combine.
4. Serve immediately or chill for an hour to let flavors meld.

TIPS:

- For a less spicy salad, remove the jalapeño seeds and membrane.
- Add corn for a sweet contrast to the spicy jalapeño.

N.V.: Calories: 350, Fat: 15g, Carbs: 42g, Protein: 12g, Sugar: 3g

ASIAN CHICKEN SALAD WITH GINGER DRESSING

PREPARATION TIME: 20 min - **COOKING TIME:** 0 min **MODE OF COOKING:** Assembling - **SERVINGS:** 2 **INGREDIENTS:**

- 2 cups shredded cooked chicken breast
- 2 cups shredded cabbage (mix of red and green)
- 1 carrot, julienned
- 1/2 cucumber, julienned
- 1/4 cup sliced almonds
- 1/4 cup fresh cilantro, chopped
- 2 Tbsp sesame seeds
- **For the dressing:**
  - 1/4 cup olive oil
  - 2 Tbsp soy sauce
  - 1 Tbsp rice vinegar
  - 1 Tbsp fresh ginger, grated
  - 1 tsp honey
  - 1 garlic clove, minced

DIRECTIONS:

1. In a large bowl, combine shredded chicken, cabbage, carrot, cucumber, almonds, cilantro, and sesame seeds.
2. In a small bowl, whisk together all dressing ingredients until well combined.
3. Drizzle the dressing over the salad and toss to coat evenly.
4. Serve immediately or let sit for 10 minutes to allow flavors to meld.

TIPS:

- For a vegetarian version, replace chicken with tofu or edamame.
- Add mandarin orange segments for a sweet citrus note.

N.V.: Calories: 400, Fat: 25g, Carbs: 18g, Protein: 27g, Sugar: 5g

MEDITERRANEAN LENTIL SALAD

PREPARATION TIME: 15 min - **COOKING TIME:** 0 min (assuming pre-cooked lentils) **MODE OF COOKING:** Assembling - **SERVINGS:** 2 **INGREDIENTS:**

- 2 cups cooked lentils
- 1/2 cup cherry tomatoes, halved
- 1/2 cucumber, diced
- 1/4 red onion, thinly sliced
- 1/4 cup kalamata olives, halved
- 1/4 cup feta cheese, crumbled
- **For the dressing:**
  - 3 Tbsp olive oil
  - 1 Tbsp lemon juice
  - 1 tsp dried oregano
  - Salt and pepper to taste

DIRECTIONS:

1. In a large bowl, mix together lentils, cherry tomatoes, cucumber, red onion, olives, and feta cheese.
2. In a small bowl, whisk together olive oil, lemon juice, oregano, salt, and pepper.
3. Pour dressing over salad and toss to combine.
4. Chill for at least 30 minutes before serving to enhance flavors.

TIPS:

- Serve over a bed of fresh spinach for extra greens.
- Drizzle with a little more olive oil before serving for added richness.

N.V.: Calories: 360, Fat: 20g, Carbs: 32g, Protein: 14g, Sugar: 5g

WATERMELON AND FETA SALAD WITH MINT

PREPARATION TIME: 10 min - **COOKING TIME:** 0 min **MODE OF COOKING:** Assembling - **SERVINGS: 2 INGREDIENTS:**
- 3 cups cubed watermelon
- 1/2 cup feta cheese, cubed or crumbled
- 1/4 cup fresh mint leaves, chopped
- 2 Tbsp balsamic glaze

DIRECTIONS:
1. In a large bowl, combine watermelon, feta, and mint.
2. Drizzle with balsamic glaze just before serving.
3. Gently toss to combine.

TIPS:
- Chill the watermelon beforehand for a refreshing summer dish.
- Add thinly sliced red onion for a sharp contrast in flavor.

N.V.: Calories: 180, Fat: 7g, Carbs: 27g, Protein: 5g, Sugar: 22g

CRUNCHY CABBAGE AND CARROT SLAW

PREPARATION TIME: 15 min - **COOKING TIME:** 0 min **MODE OF COOKING:** Assembling - **SERVINGS: 2 INGREDIENTS:**
- 2 cups shredded red cabbage
- 1 cup shredded carrots
- 1/4 cup chopped fresh cilantro
- 1/4 cup toasted sesame seeds
- **For the dressing:**
  - 3 Tbsp apple cider vinegar
  - 2 Tbsp honey
  - 1 Tbsp sesame oil
  - Salt and pepper to taste

DIRECTIONS:
1. In a large bowl, combine shredded cabbage, carrots, and cilantro.
2. In a small bowl, whisk together apple cider vinegar, honey, sesame oil, salt, and pepper to create the dressing.
3. Pour the dressing over the cabbage mixture and toss thoroughly to coat.
4. Sprinkle toasted sesame seeds over the top before serving.

TIPS:
- Allow the slaw to marinate for at least 30 minutes before serving to enhance the flavors.
- Add chopped nuts like almonds or peanuts for an extra crunch.

AVOCADO AND SHRIMP SALAD

PREPARATION TIME: 15 min - **COOKING TIME:** 0 min **MODE OF COOKING:** Assembling - **SERVINGS: 2 INGREDIENTS:**
- 1 cup cooked shrimp, peeled and deveined
- 1 ripe avocado, diced
- 1/2 cucumber, diced
- 1/4 red onion, thinly sliced
- 1/2 cup cherry tomatoes, halved
- 1/4 cup fresh cilantro, chopped

- **For the dressing:**
  - Juice of 1 lime
  - 2 Tbsp extra virgin olive oil
  - 1 garlic clove, minced
  - Salt and pepper to taste

DIRECTIONS:
1. In a large bowl, combine shrimp, avocado, cucumber, red onion, cherry tomatoes, and cilantro.
2. In a small bowl, whisk together lime juice, olive oil, minced garlic, salt, and pepper to create the dressing.
3. Drizzle the dressing over the salad ingredients and gently toss to coat evenly.
4. Chill for about 10 minutes before serving to allow the flavors to meld.

TIPS:
- Ensure the shrimp are well-drained to prevent the salad from becoming watery.
- For an extra kick, add a pinch of chili flakes to the dressing.

N.V.: Calories: 290, Fat: 20g, Carbs: 12g, Protein: 17g, Sugar: 2g

6.2 WARM SOUP RECIPES FOR ANY SEASON

Soups are a comforting staple for any season, especially for women over 50 who can benefit from the nutrient-rich, hydrating qualities of a well-prepared broth. Each recipe in this selection is designed with health in mind, focusing on metabolic boosters, high-fiber content, and ingredients known for their supportive role in hormonal balance and inflammation reduction. From light, refreshing summer soups to hearty, warming winter bowls, these dishes are perfect for incorporating into an intermittent fasting regimen, providing satisfaction without heaviness. The recipes vary in flavors, utilizing seasonal vegetables and lean proteins, ensuring that there's a delightful soup for any palate or dietary need.

ROASTED TOMATO AND BASIL SOUP

PREPARATION TIME: 10 min - **COOKING TIME:** 50 min
MODE OF COOKING: Roasting and Simmering - **SERVINGS:** 4
INGREDIENTS:
- 3 lb tomatoes, halved
- 4 Tbsp olive oil
- Salt and pepper to taste
- 1 onion, diced
- 2 cloves garlic, minced
- 2 cups vegetable broth
- 2 tsp balsamic vinegar
- 1/2 cup fresh basil leaves, chopped

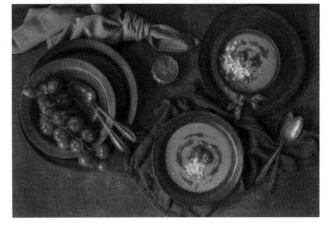

DIRECTIONS:
1. Preheat oven to 425°F (218°C). Place tomatoes on a baking sheet, drizzle with 2 Tbsp olive oil, and season with salt and pepper. Roast until caramelized, about 40 min.
2. In a large pot, heat the remaining 2 Tbsp olive oil over medium heat. Add onion and garlic, sauté until softened.
3. Add roasted tomatoes, vegetable broth, and balsamic vinegar. Bring to a simmer and cook for 10 min.
4. Remove from heat, add basil, and blend until smooth.
5. Return to the pot, adjust seasoning, and heat through before serving.

TIPS:
- Serve with a dollop of Greek yogurt for added creaminess.
- Pair with a slice of whole-grain bread for a complete meal.

N.V.: Calories: 178, Fat: 10g, Carbs: 20g, Protein: 3g, Sugar: 12g

SPICED CARROT AND GINGER SOUP

PREPARATION TIME: 15 min - **COOKING TIME:** 30 min
MODE OF COOKING: Simmering - **SERVINGS:** 4
INGREDIENTS:
- 2 Tbsp olive oil
- 1 onion, chopped
- 4 cups carrots, peeled and diced
- 3 Tbsp fresh ginger, minced
- 4 cups vegetable broth
- 1 tsp ground cumin
- 1 tsp ground coriander
- Salt and pepper to taste
- 1 cup light coconut milk

DIRECTIONS:
1. Heat olive oil in a large pot over medium heat. Add onion and sauté until translucent.
2. Add carrots and ginger, cooking for another 5 min.
3. Stir in cumin and coriander, cooking for 1 min until fragrant.
4. Pour in vegetable broth and bring to a boil. Reduce heat and simmer until carrots are tender, about 20 min.
5. Blend the soup in batches in a blender or use an immersion blender until smooth.
6. Return to pot, stir in coconut milk, and heat through. Adjust seasoning with salt and pepper.

TIPS:
- Garnish with a swirl of coconut milk and a sprinkle of chopped cilantro for an extra touch of flavor.
- Add a pinch of chili flakes for a spicy kick.

N.V.: Calories: 200, Fat: 9g, Carbs: 27g, Protein: 3g, Sugar: 13g

ROASTED TOMATO AND BASIL SOUP

PREPARATION TIME: 10 min - **COOKING TIME:** 50 min
MODE OF COOKING: Roasting and Simmering - **SERVINGS:** 4
INGREDIENTS:
- 3 lb tomatoes, halved
- 4 Tbsp olive oil
- Salt and pepper to taste
- 1 onion, diced
- 2 cloves garlic, minced
- 2 cups vegetable broth
- 2 tsp balsamic vinegar
- 1/2 cup fresh basil leaves, chopped

DIRECTIONS:
1. Preheat oven to 425°F (218°C). Place tomatoes on a baking sheet, drizzle with 2 Tbsp olive oil, and season with salt and pepper. Roast until caramelized, about 40 min.
2. In a large pot, heat the remaining 2 Tbsp olive oil over medium heat. Add onion and garlic, sauté until softened.
3. Add roasted tomatoes, vegetable broth, and balsamic vinegar. Bring to a simmer and cook for 10 min.
4. Remove from heat, add basil, and blend until smooth.
5. Return to the pot, adjust seasoning, and heat through before serving.

TIPS:
- Serve with a dollop of Greek yogurt for added creaminess.
- Pair with a slice of whole-grain bread for a complete meal.

N.V.: Calories: 178, Fat: 10g, Carbs: 20g, Protein: 3g, Sugar: 12g

CREAMY ASPARAGUS SOUP

PREPARATION TIME: 10 min - **COOKING TIME:** 20 min
MODE OF COOKING: Blending and Simmering - **SERVINGS:** 4
INGREDIENTS:
- 1 Tbsp olive oil
- 1 shallot, chopped
- 2 bunches asparagus, trimmed and cut into 1-inch pieces
- 3 cups low-sodium vegetable broth
- Salt and pepper to taste
- 1/2 cup low-fat Greek yogurt

DIRECTIONS:
1. Heat olive oil in a large pot over medium heat. Add shallot and sauté until translucent.
2. Add asparagus and cook for 5 min, stirring occasionally.
3. Pour in vegetable broth, bring to a boil, then reduce heat and simmer until asparagus is very tender, about 15 min.
4. Remove from heat, blend until smooth using an immersion blender or in batches with a standard blender.
5. Stir in Greek yogurt until well combined and season with salt and pepper. Serve warm.

TIPS:
- Enhance the flavor with a squeeze of lemon juice just before serving.
- For a richer texture, substitute Greek yogurt with light cream.

N.V.: Calories: 98, Fat: 4g, Carbs: 12g, Protein: 6g, Sugar: 5g

WHITE BEAN AND KALE SOUP

PREPARATION TIME: 15 min - **COOKING TIME:** 40 min
MODE OF COOKING: Simmering - **SERVINGS:** 4
INGREDIENTS:
- 2 Tbsp olive oil
- 1 onion, diced
- 2 carrots, diced
- 2 stalks celery, diced
- 4 cloves garlic, minced
- 1 qt vegetable broth
- 1 can (15 oz) white beans, drained and rinsed
- 1 tsp dried thyme
- 1 bunch kale, stems removed and leaves chopped
- Salt and pepper to taste

DIRECTIONS:
1. Heat olive oil in a large pot over medium heat. Add onion, carrots, celery, and garlic. Sauté until vegetables are softened.
2. Add vegetable broth, white beans, and thyme. Bring to a boil, then reduce heat and simmer for 30 min.
3. Stir in kale and cook until wilted, about 10 min. Season with salt and pepper.

TIPS:
- Add a parmesan rind during simmering for extra umami flavor.
- Serve with crusty whole-grain bread for dipping.

N.V.: Calories: 245, Fat: 7g, Carbs: 35g, Protein: 12g, Sugar: 4g

MISO MUSHROOM SOUP

PREPARATION TIME: 10 min - **COOKING TIME:** 20 min
MODE OF COOKING: Simmering - **SERVINGS:** 4
INGREDIENTS:
- 2 Tbsp sesame oil
- 1 onion, sliced
- 2 cups assorted mushrooms, sliced (shiitake, button, cremini)
- 4 Tbsp miso paste
- 4 cups vegetable broth
- 1 Tbsp soy sauce
- 1 tsp ginger, grated
- 2 scallions, thinly sliced

DIRECTIONS:
1. Heat sesame oil in a pot over medium heat. Add onion and sauté until translucent.
2. Add mushrooms and cook until they begin to soften.
3. In a small bowl, dissolve miso pastes in a bit of the vegetable broth to make a smooth mixture.
4. Add the remaining broth, soy sauce, and ginger to the pot. Stir in the miso mixture. Bring to a simmer and cook for 15 min.
5. Garnish with scallions before serving.

TIPS:
- Avoid boiling the soup after adding miso to preserve its health benefits.
- Serve with a drizzle of toasted sesame oil for an extra depth of flavor.

N.V.: Calories: 110, Fat: 7g, Carbs: 10g, Protein: 3g, Sugar: 5g

SWEET POTATO AND LENTIL SOUP

PREPARATION TIME: 15 min - **COOKING TIME:** 40 min
MODE OF COOKING: Simmering - **SERVINGS:** 4
INGREDIENTS:
- 1 Tbsp olive oil
- 1 onion, chopped
- 2 cloves garlic, minced
- 1 tsp ground cumin
- 1 tsp smoked paprika
- 3 cups vegetable broth
- 1 large sweet potato, peeled and diced
- 1 cup red lentils, rinsed
- Salt and pepper to taste
- Fresh cilantro, for garnish

DIRECTIONS:
1. Heat olive oil in a large pot over medium heat. Add onion and garlic, sauté until onion is translucent.
2. Stir in cumin and smoked paprika, cook for 1 min until fragrant.
3. Add vegetable broth, sweet potatoes, and lentils. Bring to a boil, then reduce heat and simmer until sweet potatoes and lentils are tender, about 30 min.
4. Season with salt and pepper. Serve hot, garnished with fresh cilantro.

TIPS:
- For a creamier texture, blend half of the soup and then mix back into the pot.
- Serve with a slice of rustic bread for a filling meal.

N.V.: Calories: 235, Fat: 4g, Carbs: 39g, Protein: 12g, Sugar: 6g

ZUCCHINI BASIL SOUP

PREPARATION TIME: 10 min - **COOKING TIME:** 20 min
MODE OF COOKING: Blending and Simmering - **SERVINGS:** 4
INGREDIENTS:
- 2 Tbsp olive oil
- 2 medium zucchinis, sliced
- 1 onion, chopped
- 2 cloves garlic, minced
- 4 cups vegetable broth
- 1/2 cup fresh basil leaves
- Salt and pepper to taste
- 1/4 cup grated Parmesan cheese (optional)

DIRECTIONS:
1. Heat olive oil in a pot over medium heat. Add onion and garlic, cook until soft.
2. Add zucchinis and sauté for a few minutes until slightly softened.
3. Add vegetable broth and bring to a boil. Reduce heat and simmer for 10 min until zucchini is tender.
4. Remove from heat. Add basil, then blend the soup until smooth.
5. Return to pot, season with salt and pepper, and warm through. Serve garnished with grated Parmesan if desired.

TIPS:
- For a vegan option, omit Parmesan or substitute with nutritional yeast for a cheesy flavor.
- This soup is particularly refreshing in the summer, served chilled.

N.V.: Calories: 123, Fat: 7g, Carbs: 12g, Protein: 3g, Sugar: 6g

PUMPKIN GINGER SOUP

PREPARATION TIME: 10 min - **COOKING TIME:** 25 min
MODE OF COOKING: Simmering - **SERVINGS:** 4
INGREDIENTS:
- 2 Tbsp olive oil
- 1 onion, diced
- 2 Tbsp fresh ginger, minced
- 4 cups pumpkin puree (canned or homemade)
- 4 cups vegetable broth
- 1 tsp cinnamon
- 1/2 tsp nutmeg
- Salt and pepper to taste
- 1/4 cup coconut milk

DIRECTIONS:
1. Heat olive oil in a pot over medium heat. Add onion and ginger and cook until onion is translucent.
2. Add pumpkin puree, vegetable broth, cinnamon, and nutmeg. Bring to a simmer and cook for 20 min, stirring occasionally.
3. Stir in coconut milk, season with salt and pepper, and heat through. Serve warm.

TIPS:
- Enhance the flavor by roasting fresh pumpkin instead of using canned puree.
- Top with roasted pumpkin seeds for added texture and flavor.

N.V.: Calories: 140, Fat: 7g, Carbs: 18g, Protein: 2g, Sugar: 8g

6.3 LIGHT SANDWICHES AND WRAPS

Light sandwiches and wraps are perfect for incorporating into an intermittent fasting regimen, especially for women over 50 who need nutrient-dense, easy-to-digest meals. These recipes are designed to be both satisfying and healthful, supporting metabolic health and weight management. They feature lean proteins, plenty of vegetables, and whole grains, ensuring a balance of carbs, proteins, and healthy fats. Each recipe is easy to prepare and perfect for a quick lunch or a light dinner, offering versatility and flavor that can be enjoyed year-round.

TURKEY AND AVOCADO WRAP

PREPARATION TIME: 10 min - **COOKING TIME:** 0 min
MODE OF COOKING: No cook - **SERVINGS:** 4
INGREDIENTS:
- 4 whole grain wraps
- 8 oz. sliced turkey breast
- 1 ripe avocado, sliced
- 1 cup mixed salad greens
- 1/4 cup low-fat Greek yogurt
- 2 tsp Dijon mustard
- Salt and pepper to taste

DIRECTIONS:
1. Lay out the wraps on a clean surface.
2. Spread each wrap with Greek yogurt and a thin layer of Dijon mustard.
3. Layer the turkey slices evenly among the wraps, topped with avocado slices and salad greens.
4. Season with salt and pepper, then roll up the wraps tightly, slicing in half before serving.

TIPS:
- Add a sprinkle of chia seeds for extra fiber and omega-3s.
- For a gluten-free option, use gluten-free wraps.

N.V.: Calories: 270, Fat: 9g, Carbs: 27g, Protein: 20g, Sugar: 3g

CHICKEN CAESAR SALAD WRAP

PREPARATION TIME: 15 min - **COOKING TIME:** 0 min
MODE OF COOKING: No cook - **SERVINGS:** 4
INGREDIENTS:
- 4 whole grain wraps
- 2 cups cooked chicken breast, shredded
- 1 cup romaine lettuce, chopped
- 1/4 cup Parmesan cheese, shaved
- 1/4 cup Caesar dressing, low-fat
- Black pepper to taste

DIRECTIONS:
1. Lay each wrap flat on a clean surface.
2. Distribute the lettuce, chicken, and Parmesan cheese evenly among the wraps.
3. Drizzle with Caesar dressing and add a sprinkle of black pepper.
4. Roll up the wraps tightly, slicing in half before serving.

TIPS:
- For added crunch, include croutons or chopped raw vegetables.
- Opt for a yogurt-based Caesar dressing to reduce fat content.

N.V.: Calories: 320, Fat: 12g, Carbs: 28g, Protein: 25g, Sugar: 4g

SMOKED SALMON AND CREAM CHEESE BAGEL

PREPARATION TIME: 5 min - **COOKING TIME:** 0 min
MODE OF COOKING: No cook - **SERVINGS:** 4
INGREDIENTS:
- 4 whole grain bagels, halved
- 4 oz. low-fat cream cheese
- 8 oz. smoked salmon
- 1 small red onion, thinly sliced
- 1 tbsp capers
- 2 tsp fresh dill, chopped
- Freshly ground black pepper to taste

DIRECTIONS:
1. Spread each bagel half with cream cheese.
2. Layer on smoked salmon, red onion slices, and capers.
3. Sprinkle with fresh dill and black pepper.
4. Serve immediately or cover and refrigerate until serving.

TIPS:
- Toast the bagels lightly before assembling for added crunch and warmth.
- Squeeze a bit of lemon juice over the salmon for an extra zest.

N.V.: Calories: 360, Fat: 12g, Carbs: 42g, Protein: 22g, Sugar: 6g

MEDITERRANEAN VEGETABLE WRAP

PREPARATION TIME: 15 min - **COOKING TIME:** 0 min
MODE OF COOKING: No cook - **SERVINGS:** 4
INGREDIENTS:
- 4 whole wheat wraps
- 1 cup hummus
- 1 red bell pepper, sliced
- 1 zucchini, thinly sliced
- 1/2 cup feta cheese, crumbled
- 1/2 cup kalamata olives, pitted and halved
- 1 cup spinach leaves
- 1 tbsp olive oil
- Salt and pepper to taste

DIRECTIONS:
1. Spread hummus on each wrap, covering the surface.
2. Layer red bell pepper, zucchini, feta cheese, olives, and spinach leave evenly among the wraps.
3. Drizzle with olive oil and season with salt and pepper.
4. Roll the wraps tightly and slice in half before serving.

TIPS:
- For added flavor, grill the zucchini and red pepper before assembling the wraps.
- Serve with a side of Greek yogurt for dipping.

N.V.: Calories: 310, Fat: 15g, Carbs: 33g, Protein: 12g, Sugar: 5g

ROAST BEEF AND HORSERADISH CREAM WRAP

PREPARATION TIME: 10 min - **COOKING TIME:** 0 min
MODE OF COOKING: No cook - **SERVINGS:** 4
INGREDIENTS:
- 4 whole wheat wraps
- 8 oz. thinly sliced roast beef

- 1/4 cup low-fat sour cream
- 1 tbsp horseradish
- 1/2 cup arugula
- 1/4 cup red onion, thinly sliced
- Salt and pepper to taste

DIRECTIONS:
1. Mix sour cream and horseradish in a small bowl.
2. Lay out the wraps and spread each with the horseradish cream.
3. Arrange roast beef, arugula, and red onion slices evenly among the wraps.
4. Season with salt and pepper, roll up tightly, and slice in half before serving.

TIPS:
- Opt for a low-sodium roast beef to keep salt intake in check.
- Add sliced tomatoes for extra juiciness and flavor.

N.V.: Calories: 280, Fat: 9g, Carbs: 27g, Protein: 21g, Sugar: 3g

GRILLED VEGETABLE AND GOAT CHEESE PANINI

PREPARATION TIME: 15 min - **COOKING TIME:** 10 min
MODE OF COOKING: Grilling - **SERVINGS:** 4
INGREDIENTS:
- 1 zucchini, sliced lengthwise
- 1 yellow squash, sliced lengthwise
- 1 red bell pepper, seeded and sliced
- 1 eggplant, sliced into rounds
- 2 Tbsp olive oil
- Salt and pepper to taste
- 8 slices whole grain bread
- 4 oz. goat cheese, softened
- Fresh basil leaves

DIRECTIONS:
1. Brush zucchini, squash, bell pepper, and eggplant slices with olive oil and season with salt and pepper.
2. Grill vegetables on medium heat until tender and charred, about 5 min per side.
3. Spread goat cheese on four slices of bread. Layer grilled vegetables and basil leaves over the cheese. Top with another slice of bread.
4. Grill the sandwiches in a panini press or on a skillet until the bread is toasted and the cheese is melted, about 5 min on each side.

TIPS:
- Add a drizzle of balsamic glaze on the vegetables for extra flavor.
- Press the sandwich using a heavy skillet if you do not have a panini press.

N.V.: Calories: 320, Fat: 16g, Carbs: 35g, Protein: 12g, Sugar: 8g

CURRIED CHICKEN SALAD WRAP

PREPARATION TIME: 20 min - **COOKING TIME:** 0 min
MODE OF COOKING: No cook - **SERVINGS:** 4
INGREDIENTS:
- 2 cups cooked chicken breast, shredded
- 1/2 cup plain low-fat yogurt
- 2 Tbsp curry powder
- 1 apple, cored and chopped
- 1/4 cup raisins
- 1/4 cup almonds, sliced

- 4 whole wheat wraps
- 1 cup baby spinach

DIRECTIONS:

1. In a large bowl, mix the yogurt and curry powder until smooth.
2. Add the chicken, apple, raisins, and almonds to the yogurt mixture and stir to coat well.
3. Lay out the wraps and place a layer of baby spinach on each.
4. Spoon the chicken salad onto the spinach. Roll up the wraps tightly and slice in half before serving.

TIPS:

- Adjust the amount of curry powder to suit your taste for more or less spice.
- Serve chilled for a refreshing lunch option.

N.V.: Calories: 290, Fat: 8g, Carbs: 28g, Protein: 26g, Sugar: 10g

TUNA AND WHITE BEAN SALAD WRAP

PREPARATION TIME: 10 min - **COOKING TIME:** 0 min
MODE OF COOKING: No cook - **SERVINGS:** 4
INGREDIENTS:

- 1 can (6 oz) tuna, drained and flaked
- 1 can (15 oz) white beans, rinsed and drained
- 1 small red onion, finely chopped
- 1 celery stalk, chopped
- 2 Tbsp olive oil
- 1 Tbsp lemon juice
- Salt and pepper to taste
- 4 whole wheat wraps
- 1 cup arugula

DIRECTIONS:

1. In a bowl, combine tuna, white beans, red onion, celery, olive oil, and lemon juice. Season with salt and pepper to taste.
2. Lay out the wraps and place a layer of arugula on each.
3. Spoon the tuna and bean salad over the arugula. Roll up the wraps tightly and slice in half before serving.

TIPS:

- Add chopped fresh herbs like parsley or basil for extra freshness.
- For a lighter version, substitute Greek yogurt for olive oil.

N.V.: Calories: 350, Fat: 10g, Carbs: 40g, Protein: 25g, Sugar: 2g

CHAPTER 7: DINNER RECIPES

As the sun dips below the horizon and the day's bustling activities slow to a peaceful lull, dinner time becomes a cherished moment for rejuvenation and connection. In this chapter, we delve into the art of crafting evening meals that not only nourish the body but also enrich the soul, especially designed for women over 50 who embrace intermittent fasting. This transformative dietary approach doesn't just end with what you exclude during fasting windows; it's equally about what you include during your eating periods.

Our dinners are designed to complement the metabolic and hormonal needs of aging gracefully. They pivot on the balance of macronutrients to support sustained energy levels, lean muscle mass, and optimal hormonal balance. Each recipe is a symphony of flavors, carefully orchestrated to ensure that every meal is as delightful to the palate as it is beneficial to the body. Imagine dishes that combine the rich, comforting textures of proteins with the bold, antioxidative power of colorful vegetables, all spiced with herbs that whisper tales of distant lands.

Moreover, these recipes cater to the practicalities of modern life. Whether you're dining alone, with a partner, or hosting friends and family, the meals are designed to be straightforward, with ingredients that are as accessible as they are healthful. Picture yourself preparing a heart-healthy fish dish that recalls the freshness of the sea, or a plant-based dinner that celebrates the earth's bounty. Perhaps you'll find comfort in a low-carb meal that satisfies without weighing you down.

As we explore these recipes, we do so with the understanding that dinner is more than just a meal—it's a daily milestone that offers a moment to reflect, to appreciate, and to nourish not just the physical body but also the spirit. These meals are more than food; they are a ritual of self-care and a celebration of life beyond 50. With each recipe, we embrace the joy of cooking and the pleasure of eating, ensuring that each dinner enriches your journey through intermittent fasting and life's golden years.

7.1 HEART-HEALTHY FISH AND POULTRY DISHES

Fish and poultry are not only versatile ingredients but also heart-healthy options that can play a crucial role in the diet of women over 50. Rich in essential nutrients and typically lower in fat, these proteins support cardiovascular health and aid in maintaining muscle mass, which is critical during the golden years. In this sub-chapter, we explore a variety of dishes that showcase the delicate flavors and beneficial properties of fish and poultry, each recipe tailored to be both nourishing and satisfying. These dishes are crafted to be simple yet elegant, suitable for a quiet dinner at home or a festive gathering, always keeping health and enjoyment hand in hand.

LEMON HERB BAKED SALMON

PREPARATION TIME: 10 min - **COOKING TIME:** 20 min
MODE OF COOKING: Baking - **SERVINGS:** 4
INGREDIENTS:

- 4 salmon fillets (6 oz each)
- 2 lemons, one juiced and one sliced
- 2 Tbsp olive oil
- 1 tsp dried dill
- 1 tsp dried parsley
- Salt and pepper to taste

DIRECTIONS:

1. Preheat oven to 375°F (190°C). Line a baking sheet with foil.
2. Place salmon fillets on the foil. Drizzle with olive oil and lemon juice.
3. Season with dill, parsley, salt, and pepper. Top each fillet with lemon slices.
4. Bake in the preheated oven until salmon is flaky and cooked through, about 20 min.

TIPS:
- Serve with steamed asparagus or green beans for a complete meal.
- Garnish with fresh parsley for added freshness and color.

N.V.: Calories: 295, Fat: 18g, Carbs: 3g, Protein: 30g, Sugar: 1g

TURKEY STUFFED PEPPERS

PREPARATION TIME: 20 min - **COOKING TIME:** 30 min
MODE OF COOKING: Baking - **SERVINGS:** 4
INGREDIENTS:
- 4 large bell peppers, tops cut, seeded
- 1 lb ground turkey
- 1 onion, diced
- 1 cup cooked quinoa
- 1 cup chopped tomatoes
- 1 tsp garlic powder
- 1 tsp smoked paprika
- 1/2 cup shredded low-fat mozzarella cheese
- Salt and pepper to taste

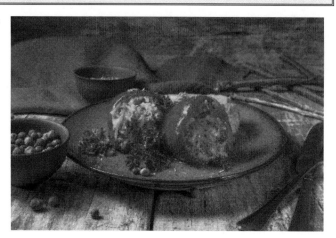

DIRECTIONS:
1. Preheat oven to 375°F (190°C).
2. In a skillet, cook ground turkey and onion over medium heat until turkey is browned.
3. Stir in quinoa, tomatoes, garlic powder, smoked paprika, salt, and pepper.
4. Stuff the mixture into the prepared peppers. Top with shredded mozzarella.
5. Bake in the preheated oven until peppers are tender and cheese is melted, about 30 min.

TIPS:
- Add a spoonful of low-fat Greek yogurt on top before serving for extra creaminess.
- Mix in some chopped spinach with the turkey for added nutrients.

N.V.: Calories: 350, Fat: 12g, Carbs: 27g, Protein: 31g, Sugar: 8g

CHICKEN PICCATA

PREPARATION TIME: 15 min - **COOKING TIME:** 20 min
MODE OF COOKING: Sautéing - **SERVINGS:** 4
INGREDIENTS:
- 4 boneless, skinless chicken breasts, pounded to even thickness
- 1/4 cup all-purpose flour (or almond flour for a lower carb option)
- 2 Tbsp olive oil
- 1/4 cup fresh lemon juice
- 1/2 cup chicken broth
- 1/4 cup capers, drained
- 2 Tbsp unsalted butter
- Salt and pepper to taste
- Chopped parsley, for garnish

DIRECTIONS:
1. Season the chicken breasts with salt and pepper, then dredge in flour to coat lightly.
2. Heat olive oil in a large skillet over medium-high heat. Add chicken and cook until golden on each side and cooked through, about 4-5 min per side. Remove chicken and set aside.
3. To the same skillet, add lemon juice, chicken broth, and capers. Bring to a boil, scraping up any browned bits from the pan.
4. Reduce heat and stir in butter until melted. Return chicken to the pan and simmer for 5 min.

5. Serve chicken with sauce spooned over the top and garnished with chopped parsley.

TIPS:
- Serve with a side of steamed vegetables or over a bed of zucchini noodles for a complete meal.
- For a richer flavor, add a splash of white wine to the sauce while cooking.

N.V.: Calories: 290, Fat: 15g, Carbs: 8g, Protein: 29g, Sugar: 0g

GINGER SOY GLAZED TILAPIA

PREPARATION TIME: 10 min - **COOKING TIME:** 15 min
MODE OF COOKING: Baking - **SERVINGS:** 4
INGREDIENTS:
- 4 tilapia fillets
- 2 Tbsp soy sauce
- 2 Tbsp honey
- 1 Tbsp fresh ginger, minced
- 2 cloves garlic, minced
- 1 Tbsp sesame oil
- 2 Tbsp green onions, sliced
- Sesame seeds, for garnish

DIRECTIONS:
1. Preheat oven to 375°F (190°C). Line a baking sheet with parchment paper.
2. In a small bowl, mix soy sauce, honey, ginger, garlic, and sesame oil.
3. Place tilapia fillets on the prepared baking sheet. Pour the soy mixture over the fillets.
4. Bake in the preheated oven until fish flakes easily with a fork, about 12-15 min.
5. Garnish with sliced green onions and sesame seeds before serving.

TIPS:
- For extra crispiness, broil the tilapia for the last 2-3 min of cooking.
- Serve with steamed rice or a side of stir-fried vegetables for a balanced meal.

N.V.: Calories: 235, Fat: 8g, Carbs: 12g, Protein: 28g, Sugar: 8g

ROSEMARY ORANGE ROASTED CHICKEN

PREPARATION TIME: 20 min - **COOKING TIME:** 1 hr 20 min
MODE OF COOKING: Roasting - **SERVINGS:** 4
INGREDIENTS:
- 1 whole chicken (about 4 lbs)
- 2 Tbsp olive oil
- 2 oranges, one juiced and one sliced
- 2 Tbsp fresh rosemary, chopped
- 4 cloves garlic, minced
- Salt and pepper to taste

DIRECTIONS:
1. Preheat oven to 375°F (190°C).
2. Rub the chicken all over with olive oil, then season inside and out with salt and pepper. Place rosemary, garlic, and orange slices inside the cavity.
3. Place the chicken in a roasting pan and roast in the preheated oven for 1 hr 20 min, or until the juices run clear. Baste occasionally with orange juice.
4. Let the chicken rest for 10 min before carving. Serve with the juices from the pan.

TIPS:
- For a crispier skin, increase the oven temperature to 400°F (204°C) for the last 15 min of roasting.
- Serve with roasted vegetables to soak up the delicious pan juices.

N.V.: Calories: 410, Fat: 23g, Carbs: 5g, Protein: 45g, Sugar: 3g

BALSAMIC GLAZED CHICKEN

PREPARATION TIME: 10 min - **COOKING TIME:** 25 min
MODE OF COOKING: Sautéing - **SERVINGS:** 4
INGREDIENTS:
- 4 boneless, skinless chicken breasts
- Salt and pepper to taste
- 2 Tbsp olive oil
- 1/4 cup balsamic vinegar
- 2 Tbsp honey
- 1/2 cup chicken broth
- 2 cloves garlic, minced
- 1 tsp dried thyme

DIRECTIONS:
1. Season chicken breasts with salt and pepper.
2. Heat olive oil in a skillet over medium-high heat. Add chicken and cook until golden on both sides, about 5-6 min per side. Remove chicken and set aside.
3. In the same skillet, add garlic and sauté until fragrant, about 1 min.
4. Add balsamic vinegar, honey, chicken broth, and thyme. Bring to a simmer and reduce the sauce by half, about 10 min.
5. Return chicken to the skillet and coat with the balsamic glaze. Cook for an additional 5 min to heat through.

TIPS:
- Garnish with fresh thyme or parsley before serving for added flavor and presentation.
- Serve with a side of roasted vegetables or over a bed of quinoa for a balanced meal.

N.V.: Calories: 280, Fat: 10g, Carbs: 15g, Protein: 34g, Sugar: 13g

HERB-CRUSTED COD

PREPARATION TIME: 15 min - **COOKING TIME:** 15 min
MODE OF COOKING: Baking - **SERVINGS:** 4
INGREDIENTS:
- 4 cod fillets (6 oz each)
- 2 Tbsp olive oil
- 1/4 cup breadcrumbs
- 1/4 cup grated Parmesan cheese
- 1 Tbsp fresh parsley, chopped
- 1 tsp dried oregano
- 1 clove garlic, minced
- Lemon wedges for serving
- Salt and pepper to taste

DIRECTIONS:
1. Preheat oven to 400°F (204°C). Line a baking sheet with parchment paper.
2. In a small bowl, mix breadcrumbs, Parmesan cheese, parsley, oregano, and minced garlic.
3. Brush each cod fillet with olive oil, season with salt and pepper, and press the herb breadcrumb mixture onto the top of each fillet.
4. Place on the prepared baking sheet and bake until the crust is golden and the fish flakes easily with a fork, about 15 min.
5. Serve with lemon wedges on the side.

TIPS:
- For a gluten-free option, use gluten-free breadcrumbs or finely ground almond flour.
- Enhance the flavor by adding a sprinkle of lemon zest to the breadcrumb mixture.

N.V.: Calories: 220, Fat: 9g, Carbs: 9g, Protein: 27g, Sugar: 1g

SPICY THAI BASIL CHICKEN

PREPARATION TIME: 10 min - **COOKING TIME:** 15 min
MODE OF COOKING: Stir-frying - **SERVINGS:** 4
INGREDIENTS:

- 1 lb chicken breast, thinly sliced
- 2 Tbsp vegetable oil
- 3 cloves garlic, minced
- 1 red bell pepper, sliced
- 1 onion, sliced
- 2 Tbsp soy sauce
- 1 Tbsp fish sauce
- 1 Tbsp sugar
- 1/2 cup Thai basil leaves
- 1 tsp chili flakes (adjust to taste)

DIRECTIONS:

1. Heat oil in a large skillet over medium-high heat. Add garlic and stir-fry until golden, about 1 min.
2. Add chicken and cook until it is nearly cooked through, about 5 min.
3. Add bell pepper and onion, stir-frying until just tender, about 3 min.
4. Stir in soy sauce, fish sauce, sugar, and chili flakes, cooking for another 2 min.
5. Remove from heat and stir in Thai basil leaves until wilted.

TIPS:

- Serve with steamed rice or rice noodles for a complete meal.
- Adjust the amount of chili flakes according to your spice preference.

N.V.: Calories: 235, Fat: 9g, Carbs: 12g, Protein: 26g, Sugar: 7g

7.2 PLANT-BASED DINNERS FOR BALANCED EATING

Embracing a plant-based diet is a wonderful way to enhance health, especially for women over 50. The recipes in this section are designed to deliver a balance of nutrients through whole foods, focusing on plant-based proteins, complex carbohydrates, and healthy fats. These dinners are not only hearty and satisfying but also help to manage weight, support hormonal balance, and reduce inflammation. Whether you're a seasoned vegan or simply looking to incorporate more plant-based meals into your diet, these recipes provide delicious options that cater to your health needs without compromising on taste.

QUINOA AND BLACK BEAN STUFFED PEPPERS

PREPARATION TIME: 20 min - **COOKING TIME:** 30 min
MODE OF COOKING: Baking - **SERVINGS:** 4
INGREDIENTS:

- 4 large bell peppers, halved and seeded
- 1 cup quinoa, cooked
- 1 can (15 oz) black beans, drained and rinsed
- 1 cup corn kernels, fresh or frozen
- 1/2 cup onions, chopped
- 2 cloves garlic, minced
- 1 tsp cumin
- 1 tsp chili powder
- 1/2 cup tomato sauce
- 1/2 cup shredded vegan cheese

- Salt and pepper to taste
- Fresh cilantro, chopped for garnish

DIRECTIONS:
1. Preheat oven to 375°F (190°C).
2. In a bowl, mix together quinoa, black beans, corn, onions, garlic, cumin, chili powder, and tomato sauce. Season with salt and pepper.
3. Stuff the halved peppers with the quinoa mixture and place in a baking dish.
4. Top each pepper with shredded vegan cheese.
5. Cover with foil and bake for 25 min. Remove foil and bake for an additional 5 min to melt the cheese.
6. Garnish with chopped cilantro before serving.

TIPS:
- Add diced avocado or a dollop of guacamole on top for extra creaminess and flavor.
- Spice it up with a splash of hot sauce or diced jalapeño.

N.V.: Calories: 295, Fat: 5g, Carbs: 50g, Protein: 13g, Sugar: 7g

CREAMY VEGAN MUSHROOM RISOTTO

PREPARATION TIME: 10 min - **COOKING TIME:** 25 min
MODE OF COOKING: Stirring/Simmering - **SERVINGS:** 4
INGREDIENTS:
- 1 cup Arborio rice
- 2 Tbsp olive oil
- 1 onion, finely chopped
- 2 cups mushrooms, sliced
- 4 cups vegetable broth, warm
- 1/2 cup vegan white wine
- 2 cloves garlic, minced
- 1 Tbsp nutritional yeast
- Salt and pepper to taste
- Fresh parsley, chopped for garnish

DIRECTIONS:
1. Heat olive oil in a large pan over medium heat. Add onion and garlic, sauté until translucent.
2. Add mushrooms and cook until they begin to soften.
3. Stir in Arborio rice and let it toast slightly before deglazing the pan with white wine.
4. Gradually add warm broth one ladle at a time, stirring continuously until the liquid is absorbed before adding more.
5. Once the rice is creamy and al dente, stir in nutritional yeast, season with salt and pepper.
6. Serve garnished with fresh parsley.

TIPS:
- For an extra boost of flavor, stir in a tablespoon of truffle oil before serving.
- Serve with a side of steamed green vegetables for a balanced meal.

N.V.: Calories: 350, Fat: 9g, Carbs: 55g, Protein: 8g, Sugar: 3g

SPICY THAI TOFU CURRY

PREPARATION TIME: 15 min - **COOKING TIME:** 20 min
MODE OF COOKING: Sautéing and Simmering - **SERVINGS:** 4
INGREDIENTS:

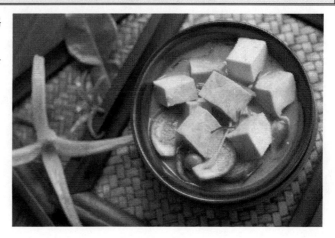

- 14 oz. firm tofu, pressed and cubed
- 1 Tbsp coconut oil
- 1 red bell pepper, sliced
- 1 zucchini, sliced
- 1 carrot, sliced
- 2 Tbsp Thai red curry paste
- 1 can (14 oz) coconut milk
- 1 Tbsp soy sauce
- 1 Tbsp brown sugar
- 1/2 cup fresh basil leaves
- Salt to taste

DIRECTIONS:

1. Heat coconut oil in a large skillet over medium heat. Add tofu and fry until golden brown on all sides, about 8 min. Remove and set aside.
2. In the same skillet, add red bell pepper, zucchini, and carrot. Sauté until they start to soften, about 5 min.
3. Stir in curry paste and cook for 1 min until fragrant.
4. Add coconut milk, soy sauce, and brown sugar. Bring to a simmer, then return the tofu to the skillet.
5. Simmer everything together for 10 min. Stir in basil leaves just before serving.

TIPS:

- Serve with jasmine rice or over quinoa for a complete meal.
- Adjust the amount of curry paste to control the level of spice.

N.V.: Calories: 330, Fat: 22g, Carbs: 20g, Protein: 15g, Sugar: 8g

WALNUT AND LENTIL BOLOGNESE

PREPARATION TIME: 20 min - **COOKING TIME:** 30 min
MODE OF COOKING: Simmering - **SERVINGS:** 4
INGREDIENTS:

- 1 cup brown lentils, cooked
- 1/2 cup walnuts, finely chopped
- 1 Tbsp olive oil
- 1 onion, chopped
- 2 cloves garlic, minced
- 1 carrot, diced
- 1 celery stalk, diced
- 1 can (14 oz) crushed tomatoes
- 1 Tbsp tomato paste
- 1 tsp dried oregano
- 1 tsp dried basil
- Salt and pepper to taste
- Fresh basil for garnish

DIRECTIONS:

1. Heat olive oil in a large pan over medium heat. Add onion, garlic, carrot, and celery, and sauté until soft, about 10 min.

2. Add walnuts and lentils, stir to combine.
3. Stir in crushed tomatoes, tomato paste, oregano, and dried basil. Simmer for 20 min, stirring occasionally.
4. Season with salt and pepper. Serve over cooked spaghetti or your favorite pasta, garnished with fresh basil.

TIPS:
- Add a splash of red wine to the sauce while cooking for added depth.
- Sprinkle with nutritional yeast before serving for a cheesy flavor.

N.V.: Calories: 295, Fat: 13g, Carbs: 33g, Protein: 12g, Sugar: 9g

ROASTED VEGETABLE AND QUINOA SALAD

PREPARATION TIME: 15 min - **COOKING TIME:** 25 min
MODE OF COOKING: Roasting - **SERVINGS:** 4
INGREDIENTS:
- 1 zucchini, cubed
- 1 bell pepper, cubed
- 1 small eggplant, cubed
- 1 red onion, chopped
- 2 Tbsp olive oil
- Salt and pepper to taste
- 1 cup quinoa, cooked
- 1/4 cup fresh parsley, chopped
- 2 Tbsp balsamic vinegar
- 1 Tbsp lemon juice

DIRECTIONS:
1. Preheat oven to 425°F (220°C).
2. Toss zucchini, bell pepper, eggplant, and red onion with olive oil, salt, and pepper. Spread on a baking sheet.
3. Roast in the preheated oven until vegetables are tender and golden, about 25 min.
4. In a large bowl, combine roasted vegetables with cooked quinoa, parsley, balsamic vinegar, and lemon juice. Toss to combine.

TIPS:
- Top with crumbled feta or goat cheese for extra flavor.
- Serve warm or at room temperature.

N.V.: Calories: 280, Fat: 10g, Carbs: 40g, Protein: 8g, Sugar: 7g

SWEET POTATO AND BLACK BEAN TACOS

PREPARATION TIME: 15 min - **COOKING TIME:** 25 min
MODE OF COOKING: Roasting - **SERVINGS:** 4
INGREDIENTS:
- 2 large sweet potatoes, peeled and diced
- 1 can (15 oz) black beans, drained and rinsed
- 2 Tbsp olive oil
- 1 tsp cumin
- 1 tsp paprika
- Salt and pepper to taste
- 8 small whole wheat tortillas
- 1 avocado, sliced
- 1/4 cup fresh cilantro, chopped
- 1 lime, cut into wedges

DIRECTIONS:

1. Preheat oven to 400°F (204°C).
2. Toss sweet potatoes with olive oil, cumin, paprika, salt, and pepper. Spread on a baking sheet and roast until tender, about 25 min.
3. Warm tortillas in the oven during the last 5 min of roasting.
4. Assemble tacos by filling each tortilla with roasted sweet potatoes, black beans, and avocado slices.
5. Garnish with fresh cilantro and serve with lime wedges.

TIPS:

- Add a dollop of vegan sour cream or a sprinkle of dairy-free cheese for extra flavor.
- Include fresh salsa or diced tomatoes for additional freshness and moisture.

N.V.: Calories: 320, Fat: 10g, Carbs: 50g, Protein: 8g, Sugar: 5g

CREAMY AVOCADO PASTA WITH PEAS

PREPARATION TIME: 10 min - **COOKING TIME:** 10 min
MODE OF COOKING: Boiling - **SERVINGS:** 4
INGREDIENTS:

- 12 oz. whole wheat pasta
- 1 ripe avocado, pitted and peeled
- 1/2 cup fresh basil leaves
- 2 cloves garlic, minced
- 2 Tbsp lemon juice
- 1/4 cup olive oil
- 1 cup green peas, frozen and thawed
- Salt and pepper to taste

DIRECTIONS:

1. Cook pasta according to package instructions until al dente. Drain, reserving 1/2 cup of the pasta water.
2. While pasta cooks, blend avocado, basil, garlic, lemon juice, and olive oil in a blender until smooth. If needed, add a little pasta water to achieve a creamy consistency.
3. Toss pasta with the avocado sauce and green peas. Season with salt and pepper.
4. Serve immediately, garnished with additional basil or vegan parmesan if desired.

TIPS:

- For a protein boost, add chickpeas or toasted pine nuts.
- Keep the pasta al dente to add texture to the creamy sauce.

N.V.: Calories: 510, Fat: 22g, Carbs: 68g, Protein: 15g, Sugar: 5g

MOROCCAN SPICED VEGGIE STEW

PREPARATION TIME: 20 min - **COOKING TIME:** 40 min
MODE OF COOKING: Simmering - **SERVINGS:** 4
INGREDIENTS:

- 1 Tbsp olive oil
- 1 onion, chopped
- 2 cloves garlic, minced
- 1 tsp ground cumin
- 1 tsp ground cinnamon
- 1 tsp ground coriander
- 1 sweet potato, peeled and cubed
- 2 carrots, peeled and sliced
- 1 zucchini, sliced
- 1 can (15 oz) diced tomatoes
- 1 can (15 oz) chickpeas, drained and rinsed

- 3 cups vegetable broth
- 1/2 cup dried apricots, chopped
- Salt and pepper to taste
- Fresh cilantro, for garnish

DIRECTIONS:
1. Heat olive oil in a large pot over medium heat. Add onion and garlic and sauté until softened.
2. Stir in cumin, cinnamon, and coriander and cook for 1 min until fragrant.
3. Add sweet potato, carrots, zucchini, diced tomatoes, chickpeas, and vegetable broth. Bring to a boil, then reduce heat and simmer for 30 min.
4. Stir in dried apricots and cook for an additional 10 min. Season with salt and pepper.
5. Serve hot, garnished with fresh cilantro.

TIPS:
- Serve this hearty stew over couscous or rice to soak up the delicious flavors.
- Add a squeeze of lemon juice before serving to enhance the flavors with a fresh zing.

N.V.: Calories: 295, Fat: 7g, Carbs: 50g, Protein: 9g, Sugar: 20g

7.3 LOW-CARB COMFORT MEALS

Embracing a low-carb lifestyle can be a fulfilling journey, especially when it involves comforting meals that satisfy both the taste buds and nutritional needs. This selection of low-carb comfort meals is crafted for those who wish to enjoy hearty flavors without the heavy load of carbohydrates. These recipes focus on maximizing taste and satisfaction by using quality proteins, healthy fats, and an array of spices and herbs to elevate each dish. Ideal for women over 50 looking to manage weight and blood sugar levels, these meals promise to nurture and nourish while keeping carb counts in check.

CAULIFLOWER RISOTTO WITH SHRIMP

PREPARATION TIME: 15 min - **COOKING TIME:** 20 min
MODE OF COOKING: Sautéing - **SERVINGS:** 4
INGREDIENTS:
- 1 large head of cauliflower, riced
- 1 lb shrimp, peeled and deveined
- 2 Tbsp olive oil
- 1 onion, finely chopped
- 2 cloves garlic, minced
- 1/2 cup chicken broth
- 1/4 cup grated Parmesan cheese
- 2 Tbsp fresh parsley, chopped
- Salt and pepper to taste

DIRECTIONS:
1. Heat olive oil in a large skillet over medium heat. Add onion and garlic, sauté until soft and translucent.
2. Add the riced cauliflower and stir to combine. Cook for about 5 min, stirring frequently.
3. Pour in chicken broth and cook until the cauliflower is tender and creamy, about 10 min.
4. Stir in the shrimp and cook until they are pink and cooked through, about 5 min.
5. Remove from heat and stir in Parmesan cheese. Season with salt and pepper to taste.
6. Garnish with fresh parsley before serving.

TIPS:
- For extra creaminess, add a splash of heavy cream or coconut milk.
- Spice it up with a pinch of red pepper flakes if desired.

N.V.: Calories: 250, Fat: 12g, Carbs: 10g, Protein: 25g, Sugar: 4g

STUFFED CHICKEN PARMESAN

PREPARATION TIME: 20 min - **COOKING TIME:** 25 min
MODE OF COOKING: Baking - **SERVINGS:** 4
INGREDIENTS:
- 4 boneless, skinless chicken breasts
- 1 cup crushed tomatoes
- 1/2 cup shredded mozzarella cheese
- 1/4 cup grated Parmesan cheese
- 2 cloves garlic, minced
- 1 tsp Italian seasoning
- Salt and pepper to taste
- 2 Tbsp olive oil

DIRECTIONS:
1. Preheat oven to 375°F (190°C).
2. Make a deep cut into each chicken breast to create a pocket.
3. Mix mozzarella, Parmesan, garlic, and Italian seasoning in a bowl. Stuff this mixture into the chicken pockets and secure with toothpicks.
4. Season chicken with salt and pepper. Heat olive oil in a skillet over medium heat and sear chicken on both sides until golden, about 3 min per side.
5. Place chicken in a baking dish, top with crushed tomatoes, and bake in the preheated oven until chicken is cooked through, about 20 min.

TIPS:
- Serve with a side of steamed vegetables or a green salad for a complete meal.
- Ensure the cheese is tucked in well to prevent it from leaking out during cooking.

N.V.: Calories: 330, Fat: 16g, Carbs: 8g, Protein: 38g, Sugar: 3g

BEEF AND BROCCOLI STIR-FRY

PREPARATION TIME: 15 min - **COOKING TIME:** 10 min
MODE OF COOKING: Stir-frying - **SERVINGS:** 4
INGREDIENTS:
- 1 lb beef sirloin, thinly sliced
- 3 cups broccoli florets
- 2 Tbsp olive oil
- 2 cloves garlic, minced
- 1 Tbsp ginger, minced
- 1/4 cup soy sauce
- 1 Tbsp sesame oil
- 1 tsp xylitol (or another sugar substitute)
- Salt and pepper to taste
- 1 Tbsp sesame seeds, for garnish

DIRECTIONS:
1. Heat olive oil in a large skillet or wok over high heat. Add garlic and ginger, and stir-fry until fragrant, about 1 min.
2. Add beef and stir-fry until it starts to brown, about 3-4 min.
3. Add broccoli and continue to stir-fry until the broccoli is tender-crisp, about 3 min.
4. In a small bowl, whisk together soy sauce, sesame oil, and xylitol. Pour over the beef and broccoli. Cook for another 2 min, allowing the sauce to thicken slightly.
5. Season with salt and pepper to taste. Garnish with sesame seeds before serving.

TIPS:
- For a complete meal, serve over cauliflower rice or alongside mixed greens.

- Add a splash of hot sauce or chili flakes for a spicy kick.

N.V.: Calories: 280, Fat: 15g, Carbs: 8g, Protein: 26g, Sugar: 2g

ZUCCHINI LASAGNA

PREPARATION TIME: 20 min - **COOKING TIME:** 45 min
MODE OF COOKING: Baking - **SERVINGS:** 6
INGREDIENTS:
- 3 large zucchinis, sliced lengthwise into thin strips
- 1 lb ground turkey
- 1 cup ricotta cheese
- 1 cup shredded mozzarella cheese
- 1/2 cup grated Parmesan cheese
- 1 can (28 oz) crushed tomatoes
- 2 cloves garlic, minced
- 1 onion, chopped
- 1 tsp dried basil
- 1 tsp dried oregano
- Salt and pepper to taste
- 2 Tbsp olive oil

DIRECTIONS:
1. Preheat oven to 375°F (190°C).
2. In a skillet, heat olive oil over medium heat. Add garlic and onion, and sauté until translucent. Add ground turkey and cook until browned.
3. Stir in crushed tomatoes, basil, oregano, salt, and pepper. Simmer for 10 min.
4. In a baking dish, layer zucchini strips, turkey tomato sauce, ricotta, mozzarella, and Parmesan. Repeat layers until all ingredients are used, finishing with cheese on top.
5. Bake in the preheated oven for 45 min, or until the top is golden and bubbly. Let stand for 10 min before serving.

TIPS:
- Pat zucchini strips with a paper towel before layering to remove excess moisture.
- For a vegetarian version, substitute ground turkey with a mix of mushrooms and spinach.

N.V.: Calories: 320, Fat: 18g, Carbs: 12g, Protein: 28g, Sugar: 6g

SPAGHETTI SQUASH WITH MEAT SAUCE

PREPARATION TIME: 10 min - **COOKING TIME:** 1 hr
MODE OF COOKING: Baking and Sautéing - **SERVINGS:** 4
INGREDIENTS:
- 1 large spaghetti squash
- 1 lb ground beef
- 2 cups tomato sauce
- 1 onion, chopped
- 2 cloves garlic, minced
- 1 Tbsp olive oil
- Salt and pepper to taste
- Fresh basil, for garnish

DIRECTIONS:
1. Preheat oven to 400°F (204°C). Halve the spaghetti squash lengthwise and scoop out the seeds. Place cut-side down on a baking sheet and bake until tender, about 40 min.

2. While the squash bakes, heat olive oil in a skillet over medium heat. Add onion and garlic, and sauté until soft. Add ground beef and cook until browned. Stir in tomato sauce and simmer until thickened, about 20 min.
3. Use a fork to scrape the spaghetti squash into strands. Top with the meat sauce.
4. Garnish with fresh basil and serve.

TIPS:
- For added flavor, mix a pinch of red pepper flakes into the meat sauce.
- Top with grated Parmesan cheese for extra richness.

N.V.: Calories: 360, Fat: 22g, Carbs: 18g, Protein: 23g, Sugar: 8g

LEMON GARLIC BUTTER SCALLOPS

PREPARATION TIME: 5 min - **COOKING TIME:** 10 min
MODE OF COOKING: Sautéing - **SERVINGS:** 4
INGREDIENTS:
- 1 lb sea scallops
- 2 Tbsp unsalted butter
- 2 cloves garlic, minced
- 1 lemon, juiced and zested
- Salt and pepper to taste
- Fresh parsley, chopped for garnish

DIRECTIONS:
1. Pat scallops dry with paper towels. Season with salt and pepper.
2. Heat a large skillet over medium-high heat. Add butter and melt until foaming.
3. Add garlic and sauté for 1 min until fragrant.
4. Add scallops to the skillet in a single layer. Cook without moving them for about 2-3 min on each side, until a golden crust forms and they are cooked through.
5. Remove from heat, drizzle with lemon juice and zest.
6. Garnish with chopped parsley before serving.

TIPS:
- Avoid overcrowding the skillet to ensure scallops get a nice sear.
- Serve over a bed of sautéed spinach or cauliflower mash for a complete low-carb meal.

N.V.: Calories: 200, Fat: 10g, Carbs: 5g, Protein: 23g, Sugar: 0g

CREAMY TUSCAN CHICKEN

PREPARATION TIME: 10 min - **COOKING TIME:** 20 min
MODE OF COOKING: Sautéing - **SERVINGS:** 4
INGREDIENTS:
- 4 boneless, skinless chicken breasts
- 1 Tbsp olive oil
- 1/2 cup sun-dried tomatoes, chopped
- 2 cloves garlic, minced
- 1 cup heavy cream
- 1/2 cup chicken broth
- 1 tsp Italian seasoning
- 1/2 cup grated Parmesan cheese
- Salt and pepper to taste
- Fresh spinach leaves

DIRECTIONS:
1. Season chicken breasts with salt and pepper.

2. Heat olive oil in a skillet over medium heat. Add chicken and cook until golden on both sides and cooked through, about 6-7 min per side. Remove chicken and set aside.
3. In the same skillet, add garlic and sun-dried tomatoes. Sauté for a few minutes until garlic is fragrant.
4. Add heavy cream, chicken broth, and Italian seasoning. Bring to a simmer.
5. Stir in Parmesan cheese until melted and sauce is creamy. Add spinach and cook until wilted.
6. Return chicken to the skillet and simmer for an additional 5 min.

TIPS:
- Serve this creamy Tuscan chicken over zucchini noodles or steamed vegetables to keep it low-carb.
- Add a splash of white wine to the sauce for added depth of flavor.

N.V.: Calories: 485, Fat: 30g, Carbs: 8g, Protein: 45g, Sugar: 4g

PORTOBELLO MUSHROOM PIZZA

PREPARATION TIME: 10 min - **COOKING TIME:** 15 min
MODE OF COOKING: Baking - **SERVINGS:** 4
INGREDIENTS:
- 4 large portobello mushroom caps, stems removed
- 1 cup marinara sauce
- 1 cup shredded mozzarella cheese
- 1/2 cup pepperoni slices
- 1 tsp dried oregano
- Salt and pepper to taste
- Olive oil for brushing

DIRECTIONS:
1. Preheat oven to 375°F (190°C).
2. Brush mushroom caps with olive oil and season with salt and pepper. Place on a baking sheet.
3. Bake for 5 min to release some moisture.
4. Remove from oven, fill each cap with marinara sauce, then top with mozzarella cheese and pepperoni slices.
5. Sprinkle oregano on top and return to the oven. Bake until the cheese is melted and bubbly, about 10 min.

TIPS:
- Customize with your favorite pizza toppings such as olives, onions, or bell peppers for more variety.
- For extra crispiness, pre-bake the mushroom caps for a longer time to ensure all moisture is released.

N.V.: Calories: 220, Fat: 14g, Carbs: 9g, Protein: 15g, Sugar: 4g

CHAPTER 8: SNACKS AND SIDES

As we navigate the journey of intermittent fasting, the importance of mindful snacking and the role of satisfying sides cannot be overstated, especially for women over 50 who are mindful of their dietary intake. Snacks and sides, often considered mere accompaniments, hold the power to transform a simple meal into a feast and an ordinary day into one brimming with zest and flavor. This chapter is dedicated to exploring those little extras that are big on nutrition and taste but still keep in line with the low-calorie, high-nutrient ethos necessary for a vibrant lifestyle.

In the spaces between meals, when hunger whispers, having a repertoire of wholesome snacks at your fingertips can make all the difference. Think of a crunchy kale chip seasoned with nutritional yeast, or a creamy hummus enriched with roasted garlic—these are not just snacks; they are mini-nutritional powerhouses that energize and satisfy without derailing your dietary goals. Similarly, the side dishes featured in this chapter are designed to complement and enhance your main meals, adding variety, color, and texture to your plate. They are thoughtfully crafted to ensure they are as nutrient-dense as they are delicious.

From vibrant, antioxidant-rich vegetable medleys that keep your plate colorful to fiber-filled legumes that pack a punch in terms of both taste and satiety, each recipe is a celebration of flavors that cater to the mature palate. And let's not forget about those low-carb indulgences that cleverly swap traditional starches with inventive, vegetable-based alternatives, ensuring that every bite provides a burst of flavor without the guilt.

As we delve into these recipes, remember that each snack and side dish has been chosen not just for its taste but for its ability to support your health and fasting goals, proving that small bites can indeed lead to big health benefits. Whether you're looking for something to tide you over until dinner or a side dish to round out a family meal, this chapter promises to enhance your culinary repertoire with options that are both nourishing and delightful.

8.1 FIBER-RICH SNACKS FOR FULLNESS

Fiber is a fundamental component of a healthy diet, especially for women over 50 who are managing their weight and enhancing their metabolic health through intermittent fasting. High-fiber snacks not only promote a feeling of fullness but also help maintain digestive health and stabilize blood sugar levels. This selection of fiber-rich snacks is designed to be both nutritious and satisfying, incorporating a variety of whole grains, nuts, seeds, and vegetables to create snacks that are as enjoyable as they are beneficial.

OAT AND BERRY ENERGY BARS

PREPARATION TIME: 15 min - **COOKING TIME:** 25 min
MODE OF COOKING: Baking - **SERVINGS:** 8
INGREDIENTS:

- 2 cups rolled oats
- 1/2 cup mixed dried berries (cranberries, blueberries, cherries)
- 1/4 cup flaxseeds
- 1/4 cup sunflower seeds
- 1/4 cup pumpkin seeds
- 1/4 cup honey
- 1/4 cup almond butter
- 1 tsp vanilla extract
- 1/2 tsp cinnamon
- Pinch of salt

DIRECTIONS:

1. Preheat oven to 350°F (175°C). Line an 8x8 inch baking pan with parchment paper.
2. In a large bowl, mix oats, dried berries, flaxseeds, sunflower seeds, and pumpkin seeds.

3. In a small saucepan, heat honey and almond butter over low heat until melted. Stir in vanilla extract, cinnamon, and salt.
4. Pour the wet ingredients over the oat mixture and stir until well combined.
5. Press the mixture firmly into the prepared pan.
6. Bake in the preheated oven for 25 min until the edges are golden brown.
7. Let cool completely before cutting into bars.

TIPS:
- Store bars in an airtight container to keep them fresh.
- Substitute any nuts or seeds you prefer to vary the flavor and texture.

N.V.: Calories: 210, Fat: 10g, Carbs: 27g, Protein: 6g, Sugar: 12g

CHICKPEA AND AVOCADO TOAST

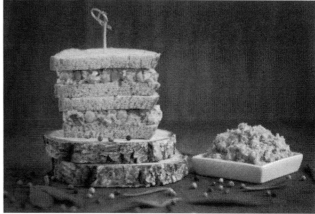

PREPARATION TIME: 10 min - **COOKING TIME:** 0 min
MODE OF COOKING: Assembly - **SERVINGS:** 4
INGREDIENTS:
- 1 can (15 oz) chickpeas, rinsed and drained
- 2 ripe avocados
- Juice of 1 lemon
- 4 slices whole-grain bread, toasted
- 1/2 tsp paprika
- Salt and pepper to taste
- Fresh cilantro, for garnish

DIRECTIONS:
1. In a bowl, mash the chickpeas and avocados together. Stir in lemon juice, paprika, salt, and pepper.
2. Spread the mixture evenly on toasted bread slices.
3. Garnish with fresh cilantro before serving.

TIPS:
- For added crunch, top with sliced radishes or cucumbers.
- Drizzle with a bit of olive oil for an extra layer of flavor.

N.V.: Calories: 290, Fat: 15g, Carbs: 34g, Protein: 10g, Sugar: 5g

SWEET POTATO HUMMUS

PREPARATION TIME: 15 min - **COOKING TIME:** 45 min
MODE OF COOKING: Baking and Blending - **SERVINGS:** 6
INGREDIENTS:
- 2 medium sweet potatoes, peeled and cubed
- 1 can (15 oz) chickpeas, drained and rinsed
- 2 cloves garlic
- 2 Tbsp tahini
- 2 Tbsp olive oil
- Juice of 1 lemon
- 1/2 tsp smoked paprika
- Salt and pepper to taste

DIRECTIONS:
1. Preheat oven to 400°F (204°C). Place sweet potato cubes on a baking sheet, drizzle with 1 Tbsp olive oil, and season with salt and pepper. Roast until tender, about 30-35 min.
2. In a food processor, combine roasted sweet potatoes, chickpeas, garlic, tahini, 1 Tbsp olive oil, lemon juice, and smoked paprika. Blend until smooth.
3. Season with salt and pepper to taste. Serve with a drizzle of olive oil and a sprinkle of paprika.

TIPS:
- Serve with a selection of raw vegetables or whole-grain crackers for dipping.
- Add more lemon juice or tahini to adjust the consistency and flavor to your liking.

N.V.: Calories: 180, Fat: 8g, Carbs: 24g, Protein: 5g, Sugar: 5g

CARROT AND APPLE SLAW

PREPARATION TIME: 10 min - **COOKING TIME:** 0 min
MODE OF COOKING: Mixing - **SERVINGS:** 4
INGREDIENTS:
- 4 large carrots, grated
- 2 apples, grated
- 1/4 cup raisins
- Juice of 1 lemon
- 2 Tbsp olive oil
- 1 Tbsp honey
- Salt and pepper to taste
- Fresh parsley, chopped for garnish

DIRECTIONS:
1. In a large bowl, combine grated carrots, apples, and raisins.
2. In a small bowl, whisk together lemon juice, olive oil, honey, salt, and pepper.
3. Pour the dressing over the carrot and apple mixture and toss to coat evenly.
4. Garnish with chopped parsley before serving.

TIPS:
- For added crunch, include chopped nuts such as walnuts or almonds.
- Chill in the refrigerator for at least an hour before serving to enhance the flavors.

N.V.: Calories: 160, Fat: 7g, Carbs: 25g, Protein: 1g, Sugar: 18g

SPINACH AND FETA STUFFED MUSHROOMS

PREPARATION TIME: 20 min - **COOKING TIME:** 15 min
MODE OF COOKING: Baking - **SERVINGS:** 4
INGREDIENTS:
- 12 large button mushrooms, stems removed
- 1 Tbsp olive oil
- 2 cups spinach, chopped
- 1/2 cup feta cheese, crumbled
- 1 clove garlic, minced
- Salt and pepper to taste
- 1/4 cup breadcrumbs

DIRECTIONS:
1. Preheat oven to 375°F (190°C).
2. In a skillet, heat olive oil over medium heat. Add garlic and sauté for 1 min. Add spinach and cook until wilted, about 3 min. Remove from heat and let cool.
3. In a bowl, mix cooked spinach, feta cheese, and breadcrumbs. Season with salt and pepper.
4. Stuff each mushroom cap with the spinach and feta mixture.
5. Place stuffed mushrooms on a baking sheet and bake in the preheated oven for 15 min or until the mushrooms are tender and the tops are golden brown.

TIPS:
- Serve as a hearty snack or alongside a main dish for a complete meal.
- For a gluten-free version, substitute breadcrumbs with gluten-free panko or almond meal.

N.V.: Calories: 150, Fat: 9g, Carbs: 10g, Protein: 6g, Sugar: 3g

EDAMAME AND CHICKPEA SALAD

PREPARATION TIME: 10 min - **COOKING TIME:** 0 min
MODE OF COOKING: Mixing - **SERVINGS:** 4
INGREDIENTS:
- 1 cup shelled edamame, cooked and cooled
- 1 can (15 oz) chickpeas, drained and rinsed
- 1 red bell pepper, diced
- 1/4 cup red onion, finely chopped
- 1/4 cup fresh cilantro, chopped
- 2 Tbsp olive oil
- Juice of 1 lime
- Salt and pepper to taste

DIRECTIONS:
1. In a large bowl, combine edamame, chickpeas, red bell pepper, red onion, and cilantro.
2. In a small bowl, whisk together olive oil, lime juice, salt, and pepper.
3. Pour the dressing over the salad and toss to coat evenly.
4. Chill in the refrigerator before serving to allow flavors to meld.

TIPS:
- Add crumbled feta or goat cheese for a creamy texture and extra flavor.
- This salad can be stored in the refrigerator for up to 3 days, making it a great make-ahead snack option.

N.V.: Calories: 220, Fat: 10g, Carbs: 25g, Protein: 10g, Sugar: 5g

ROASTED CHICKPEAS

PREPARATION TIME: 5 min - **COOKING TIME:** 30 min
MODE OF COOKING: Roasting - **SERVINGS:** 4
INGREDIENTS:
- 2 cans (15 oz each) chickpeas, drained, rinsed, and patted dry
- 2 Tbsp olive oil
- 1 tsp smoked paprika
- 1/2 tsp garlic powder
- Salt and pepper to taste

DIRECTIONS:
1. Preheat oven to 400°F (204°C).
2. In a bowl, toss the chickpeas with olive oil, smoked paprika, garlic powder, salt, and pepper.
3. Spread the chickpeas in an even layer on a baking sheet.
4. Roast in the preheated oven for 30 min, stirring occasionally, until crisp and golden.

TIPS:
- Experiment with different seasonings like curry powder or cayenne pepper for a variety of flavors.
- These make a great crunchy topping for salads or soups.

N.V.: Calories: 180, Fat: 10g, Carbs: 18g, Protein: 6g, Sugar: 0g

KALE CHIPS

PREPARATION TIME: 10 min - **COOKING TIME:** 20 min
MODE OF COOKING: Baking - **SERVINGS:** 4
INGREDIENTS:
- 1 large bunch of kale, leaves torn from stems and chopped
- 2 Tbsp olive oil
- Salt and pepper to taste

DIRECTIONS:
1. Preheat oven to 300°F (150°C).

2. In a large bowl, massage kale leaves with olive oil, then season with salt and pepper.
3. Spread kale in a single layer on a baking sheet.
4. Bake in the preheated oven until crisp, about 15-20 min, turning halfway through.

TIPS:
- Ensure kale is dry before oiling to help them crisp up.
- Add nutritional yeast before baking for a cheesy flavor without the dairy.

N.V.: Calories: 110, Fat: 7g, Carbs: 10g, Protein: 3g, Sugar: 0g

---

PEANUT BUTTER BANANA ROLLS

PREPARATION TIME: 10 min - **COOKING TIME:** 0 min
MODE OF COOKING: Assembly - **SERVINGS:** 4
INGREDIENTS:
- 4 whole wheat tortillas
- 2 bananas
- 1/4 cup natural peanut butter
- 2 Tbsp honey
- 1/4 cup granola

DIRECTIONS:
1. Spread peanut butter evenly on each tortilla.
2. Drizzle honey over the peanut butter.
3. Place a banana on each tortilla and sprinkle granola over it.
4. Roll up the tortillas tightly around the banana, then slice into bite-sized pieces.

TIPS:
- Substitute peanut butter with almond butter for a different taste.
- Add a sprinkle of cinnamon or cocoa powder for extra flavor.

N.V.: Calories: 280, Fat: 10g, Carbs: 42g, Protein: 8g, Sugar: 20g

8.2 CREATIVE SIDES TO COMPLEMENT ANY MEAL

Creative sides are essential for transforming any meal from ordinary to extraordinary. They introduce new textures, flavors, and colors that can elevate the main course, while also providing additional nutrients. This selection of side dishes focuses on using seasonal vegetables and interesting preparation techniques to bring freshness and innovation to your table. Whether paired with a hearty entrée or enjoyed on their own, these sides are designed to complement any meal and satisfy a variety of dietary preferences, making every dining experience both delicious and memorable.

ROASTED BRUSSELS SPROUTS WITH CRANBERRIES AND PECANS

PREPARATION TIME: 10 min - **COOKING TIME:** 20 min
MODE OF COOKING: Roasting - **SERVINGS:** 4
INGREDIENTS:
- 1 lb Brussels sprouts, halved
- 1/2 cup dried cranberries
- 1/2 cup pecans, roughly chopped
- 2 Tbsp olive oil
- 2 Tbsp balsamic vinegar
- Salt and pepper to taste

DIRECTIONS:
1. Preheat oven to 400°F (204°C).
2. In a large bowl, toss Brussels sprouts with olive oil, salt, and pepper. Spread on a baking sheet in a single layer.

3. Roast for 15 minutes. Add cranberries and pecans to the baking sheet, stir to combine.
4. Continue roasting for another 5 minutes or until Brussels sprouts are tender and caramelized.
5. Drizzle with balsamic vinegar before serving.

TIPS:
- For added sweetness, drizzle with a little honey along with the balsamic vinegar.
- Toast the pecans in a dry skillet prior to adding them for extra crunch.

N.V.: Calories: 220, Fat: 14g, Carbs: 22g, Protein: 4g, Sugar: 11g

CAULIFLOWER RICE TABBOULEH

PREPARATION TIME: 15 min - **COOKING TIME:** 0 min
MODE OF COOKING: Mixing - **SERVINGS:** 4
INGREDIENTS:
- 1 large head of cauliflower, riced
- 1 cup fresh parsley, finely chopped
- 1/2 cup fresh mint, finely chopped
- 1/4 cup fresh lemon juice
- 1/4 cup olive oil
- 1 cucumber, diced
- 2 tomatoes, diced
- Salt and pepper to taste

DIRECTIONS:
1. In a large bowl, combine riced cauliflower, parsley, mint, cucumber, and tomatoes.
2. In a small bowl, whisk together lemon juice, olive oil, salt, and pepper.
3. Pour the dressing over the cauliflower mixture and toss well to combine.
4. Let sit for at least 10 minutes to allow flavors to meld before serving.

TIPS:
- Chill in the refrigerator for an hour before serving to enhance the flavors.
- Add diced avocado for extra creaminess and a boost of healthy fats.

N.V.: Calories: 180, Fat: 14g, Carbs: 12g, Protein: 3g, Sugar: 5g

GARLIC PARMESAN MASHED CAULIFLOWER

PREPARATION TIME: 10 min - **COOKING TIME:** 15 min
MODE OF COOKING: Boiling and Mashing - **SERVINGS:** 4
INGREDIENTS:
- 1 large head cauliflower, cut into florets
- 3 cloves garlic, minced
- 1/4 cup grated Parmesan cheese
- 2 Tbsp unsalted butter
- 1/4 cup heavy cream
- Salt and pepper to taste

DIRECTIONS:
1. Bring a large pot of water to a boil. Add cauliflower florets and cook until very tender, about 10 min.
2. Drain well and return cauliflower to the pot. Add garlic, Parmesan, butter, and heavy cream.
3. Mash the mixture until smooth and creamy. Season with salt and pepper to taste.
4. Serve warm, garnished with additional Parmesan if desired.

TIPS:
- For a lighter version, substitute heavy cream with Greek yogurt or a splash of milk.
- Roast the garlic prior to mashing for a more mellow, sweet flavor.

N.V.: Calories: 190, Fat: 14g, Carbs: 10g, Protein: 6g, Sugar: 4g

SPICY SWEET POTATO WEDGES

PREPARATION TIME: 10 min - **COOKING TIME:** 25 min
MODE OF COOKING: Roasting - **SERVINGS:** 4
INGREDIENTS:

- 2 large sweet potatoes, cut into wedges
- 2 Tbsp olive oil
- 1 tsp smoked paprika
- 1/2 tsp cayenne pepper
- Salt and pepper to taste

DIRECTIONS:

1. Preheat oven to 425°F (220°C).
2. Toss sweet potato wedges with olive oil, smoked paprika, cayenne pepper, salt, and pepper.
3. Spread in a single layer on a baking sheet and roast until tender and crispy, about 25 min, turning halfway through.
4. Serve hot, garnished with fresh cilantro or parsley if desired.

TIPS:

- Serve with a side of avocado yogurt dip for a cooling contrast.
- For extra crispiness, allow potatoes to dry for 10 minutes after cutting and before tossing with oil and spices.

N.V.: Calories: 200, Fat: 7g, Carbs: 32g, Protein: 3g, Sugar: 7g

CREAMY CUCUMBER SALAD

PREPARATION TIME: 10 min - **COOKING TIME:** 0 min
MODE OF COOKING: Mixing - **SERVINGS:** 4
INGREDIENTS:

- 2 large cucumbers, thinly sliced
- 1/4 cup red onion, thinly sliced
- 1/2 cup Greek yogurt
- 2 Tbsp fresh dill, chopped
- 1 Tbsp white vinegar
- 1 Tbsp olive oil
- Salt and pepper to taste

DIRECTIONS:

1. In a large bowl, combine cucumbers and red onions.
2. In a separate small bowl, mix Greek yogurt, dill, vinegar, olive oil, salt, and pepper until smooth.
3. Pour the dressing over the cucumbers and onions and toss to coat evenly.
4. Chill in the refrigerator for at least 30 minutes before serving to allow flavors to meld.

TIPS:

- Add chopped garlic or a splash of lemon juice to the dressing for an extra tang.
- For a dairy-free version, use coconut yogurt or a vegan sour cream alternative.

N.V.: Calories: 90, Fat: 5g, Carbs: 8g, Protein: 2g, Sugar: 4g

GRILLED ZUCCHINI AND SQUASH WITH LEMON HERB DRESSING

PREPARATION TIME: 10 min - **COOKING TIME:** 10 min
MODE OF COOKING: Grilling - **SERVINGS:** 4
INGREDIENTS:

- 2 zucchinis, sliced lengthwise
- 2 yellow squashes, sliced lengthwise
- 2 Tbsp olive oil
- Salt and pepper to taste

- **For the Lemon Herb Dressing:**
- Juice of 1 lemon
- 1 clove garlic, minced
- 1/4 cup olive oil
- 2 Tbsp fresh parsley, chopped
- 1 Tbsp fresh basil, chopped
- Salt and pepper to taste

DIRECTIONS:
1. Preheat grill to medium-high heat.
2. Brush zucchini and squash slices with olive oil and season with salt and pepper.
3. Grill vegetables until tender and charred, about 3-4 minutes per side.
4. To make the dressing, whisk together lemon juice, garlic, olive oil, parsley, basil, salt, and pepper in a small bowl until combined.
5. Drizzle dressing over grilled vegetables before serving.

TIPS:
- Add other vegetables like bell peppers or asparagus for more variety.
- Serve alongside grilled chicken or fish for a complete meal.

N.V.: Calories: 180, Fat: 14g, Carbs: 12g, Protein: 2g, Sugar: 7g

BALSAMIC GLAZED BEETS

PREPARATION TIME: 10 min - **COOKING TIME:** 45 min
MODE OF COOKING: Roasting - **SERVINGS:** 4
INGREDIENTS:
- 4 large beets, peeled and diced
- 2 Tbsp olive oil
- 2 Tbsp balsamic vinegar
- Salt and pepper to taste
- 1 Tbsp fresh thyme, chopped

DIRECTIONS:
1. Preheat oven to 400°F (204°C).
2. In a bowl, toss the diced beets with olive oil, salt, and pepper.
3. Spread beets on a baking sheet and roast for 40 minutes, stirring halfway through.
4. Remove from oven and drizzle with balsamic vinegar and sprinkle with thyme. Toss to coat evenly.
5. Return to the oven for an additional 5 minutes to glaze.

TIPS:
- Serve as a warm side dish or allow to cool and add to salads.
- Garnish with goat cheese crumbles for added richness.

N.V.: Calories: 130, Fat: 7g, Carbs: 15g, Protein: 2g, Sugar: 11g

LEMON PARMESAN ASPARAGUS

PREPARATION TIME: 5 min - **COOKING TIME:** 10 min
MODE OF COOKING: Grilling or Roasting - **SERVINGS:** 4
INGREDIENTS:
- 1 lb asparagus, ends trimmed
- 2 Tbsp olive oil
- Juice and zest of 1 lemon
- 1/4 cup grated Parmesan cheese
- Salt and pepper to taste

DIRECTIONS:
1. Preheat grill to medium-high or oven to 400°F (204°C) if roasting.

2. In a mixing bowl, toss asparagus with olive oil, lemon juice, and zest. Season with salt and pepper.
3. Grill or roast asparagus until tender and slightly charred, about 8-10 minutes.
4. Sprinkle with Parmesan cheese while still warm.

TIPS:
- Serve immediately for best flavor and texture.
- Try adding crushed garlic to the olive oil mixture for a flavor boost.

N.V.: Calories: 110, Fat: 8g, Carbs: 5g, Protein: 5g, Sugar: 2g

8.3 SIMPLE, HEALTHY DIPS AND DRESSINGS

Dips and dressings are more than just accompaniments; they are the unsung heroes that can transform any snack or meal into an experience of flavors and textures. This section celebrates simple, healthy dips and dressings designed to complement a variety of dishes, from crunchy vegetables to grilled proteins. Each recipe is crafted to enhance your meals while staying aligned with nutritional goals, providing you with options that are as heart-healthy as they are delicious. Whether you're looking for a creamy dip for a party or a light dressing for your daily salads, these creations offer versatility and flavor without the guilt.

AVOCADO YOGURT DIP

PREPARATION TIME: 10 min - **COOKING TIME:** 0 min
MODE OF COOKING: Blending - **SERVINGS:** 4
INGREDIENTS:
- 1 ripe avocado
- 1 cup plain Greek yogurt
- Juice of 1 lime
- 1 clove garlic, minced
- Salt and pepper to taste
- 1 Tbsp chopped cilantro

DIRECTIONS:
1. In a blender or food processor, combine the avocado, Greek yogurt, lime juice, and garlic.
2. Blend until smooth. Season with salt and pepper to taste.
3. Transfer to a serving bowl and stir in chopped cilantro.

TIPS:
- Serve chilled with fresh vegetables or whole-grain crackers.
- For a spicy version, add a diced jalapeño or a dash of cayenne pepper.

N.V.: Calories: 120, Fat: 8g, Carbs: 8g, Protein: 5g, Sugar: 2g

CLASSIC HUMMUS

PREPARATION TIME: 10 min - **COOKING TIME:** 0 min
MODE OF COOKING: Blending - **SERVINGS:** 6
INGREDIENTS:
- 1 can (15 oz) chickpeas, drained and rinsed
- 1/4 cup tahini
- 1/4 cup olive oil
- Juice of 1 lemon
- 2 cloves garlic, minced
- Salt and pepper to taste
- 1/2 tsp paprika

DIRECTIONS:
1. In a food processor, combine chickpeas, tahini, olive oil, lemon juice, and garlic.
2. Blend until smooth and creamy. Season with salt and pepper.

3. Transfer to a serving bowl and sprinkle with paprika before serving.

TIPS:
- Add more lemon juice or tahini to adjust the flavor and consistency to your liking.
- Garnish with chopped parsley and drizzle with additional olive oil for a festive touch.

N.V.: Calories: 190, Fat: 14g, Carbs: 12g, Protein: 6g, Sugar: 2g

CILANTRO LIME DRESSING

PREPARATION TIME: 5 min - **COOKING TIME:** 0 min
MODE OF COOKING: Blending - **SERVINGS:** 4
INGREDIENTS:
- 1/2 cup fresh cilantro
- 1/4 cup olive oil
- Juice of 2 limes
- 1 clove garlic, minced
- 1 Tbsp honey
- Salt and pepper to taste

DIRECTIONS:
1. In a blender, combine cilantro, olive oil, lime juice, garlic, and honey.
2. Blend until smooth. Season with salt and pepper to taste.
3. Store in an airtight container in the refrigerator until ready to use.

TIPS:
- Perfect for drizzling over grilled vegetables or as a marinade for chicken or fish.
- Adjust the sweetness by adding more or less honey according to your preference.

N.V.: Calories: 130, Fat: 12g, Carbs: 6g, Protein: 0g, Sugar: 4g

GINGER SESAME DRESSING

PREPARATION TIME: 5 min - **COOKING TIME:** 0 min
MODE OF COOKING: Mixing - **SERVINGS:** 4
INGREDIENTS:
- 1/4 cup sesame oil
- 1/4 cup soy sauce
- 2 Tbsp rice vinegar
- 1 Tbsp fresh ginger, grated
- 1 clove garlic, minced
- 1 Tbsp honey
- 1 tsp sesame seeds

DIRECTIONS:
1. In a small bowl, whisk together sesame oil, soy sauce, rice vinegar, ginger, garlic, and honey until well blended.
2. Stir in sesame seeds.
3. Serve immediately or store in an airtight container in the refrigerator for up to a week.

TIPS:
- Drizzle over a crunchy Asian slaw or use as a dipping sauce for dumplings.
- For a spicier kick, add a squirt of sriracha or a pinch of crushed red pepper flakes.

N.V.: Calories: 140, Fat: 12g, Carbs: 7g, Protein: 1g, Sugar: 6g

MINT YOGURT DIP

PREPARATION TIME: 5 min - **COOKING TIME:** 0 min
MODE OF COOKING: Mixing - **SERVINGS:** 4
INGREDIENTS:

- 1 cup plain Greek yogurt
- 1/4 cup fresh mint, finely chopped
- 1 clove garlic, minced
- Juice of 1/2 lemon
- Salt and pepper to taste

DIRECTIONS:
1. In a bowl, combine Greek yogurt, mint, garlic, and lemon juice. Mix until smooth.
2. Season with salt and pepper to taste.
3. Chill in the refrigerator for at least 30 minutes before serving to allow flavors to meld.

TIPS:
- Perfect as a cooling accompaniment to spicy dishes or as a dip for grilled meats and vegetables.
- Add cucumber or diced avocado for a refreshing twist.

N.V.: Calories: 70, Fat: 2g, Carbs: 5g, Protein: 9g, Sugar: 4g

CREAMY AVOCADO DRESSING

PREPARATION TIME: 5 min - **COOKING TIME:** 0 min
MODE OF COOKING: Blending - **SERVINGS:** 4
INGREDIENTS:
- 1 ripe avocado
- 1/4 cup plain Greek yogurt
- 1 clove garlic
- Juice of 1 lime
- 1/4 cup cilantro, chopped
- Salt and pepper to taste
- Water as needed for thinning

DIRECTIONS:
1. In a blender, combine avocado, Greek yogurt, garlic, lime juice, and cilantro.
2. Blend until smooth, adding water as needed to reach desired consistency.
3. Season with salt and pepper to taste.

TIPS:
- Perfect for drizzling over taco salads or as a dip for fresh veggies.
- If not serving immediately, store in an airtight container with plastic wrap pressed directly on the surface to prevent browning.

N.V.: Calories: 110, Fat: 9g, Carbs: 6g, Protein: 2g, Sugar: 1g

BALSAMIC VINAIGRETTE

PREPARATION TIME: 5 min - **COOKING TIME:** 0 min
MODE OF COOKING: Mixing - **SERVINGS:** 4
INGREDIENTS:
- 1/4 cup balsamic vinegar
- 3/4 cup olive oil
- 1 tsp Dijon mustard
- 1 clove garlic, minced
- Salt and pepper to taste

DIRECTIONS:
1. In a small bowl, whisk together balsamic vinegar, Dijon mustard, and garlic.
2. Gradually whisk in olive oil until the dressing is emulsified.
3. Season with salt and pepper to taste.

TIPS:
- Store in a sealed container in the refrigerator for up to a week. Shake well before each use.

- Customize the flavor by adding herbs like thyme or rosemary.

N.V.: Calories: 190, Fat: 20g, Carbs: 2g, Protein: 0g, Sugar: 1g

LEMON TAHINI DRESSING

PREPARATION TIME: 5 min - **COOKING TIME:** 0 min
MODE OF COOKING: Mixing - **SERVINGS:** 4
INGREDIENTS:
- 1/3 cup tahini
- Juice of 1 lemon
- 1 clove garlic, minced
- 2 Tbsp water, or more as needed
- Salt and pepper to taste

DIRECTIONS:
1. In a bowl, whisk together tahini, lemon juice, and minced garlic.
2. Gradually add water until the dressing reaches your desired consistency.
3. Season with salt and pepper to taste.

TIPS:
- Ideal for drizzling over roasted vegetables or as a dressing for grain bowls.
- Adjust the consistency by adding more or less water depending on whether you prefer a thicker sauce or a lighter dressing.

N.V.: Calories: 160, Fat: 14g, Carbs: 5g, Protein: 3g, Sugar: 0g

CHAPTER 9: HEALTHY DESSERTS

The conclusion of a meal is often marked by a dessert, a sweet signifier of satisfaction and completion. But for those engaged in health-conscious lifestyles, particularly women over 50, dessert often becomes a source of guilt rather than pleasure. This chapter seeks to transform that perception, proving that desserts can both delight the palate and contribute to well-being. Each recipe in this collection is crafted not only to minimize guilt but to maximize health benefits—incorporating ingredients that add nutritional value without sacrificing flavor.

We explore innovative ways to use natural sweeteners, whole grains, and fresh fruits to create desserts that could be savored any day of the week without a hint of remorse. From rich, chocolatey treats that use cacao and dates for sweetness, to light, fruit-based desserts that celebrate the natural sugars of the ingredients themselves, this chapter is about finding balance and joy in every bite.

These desserts are designed to fit seamlessly into your lifestyle, whether you need a quick weekday sweet or something special for weekend entertaining. They respect your health goals while embracing the joy of eating, blurring the line between indulgence and nourishment. Each recipe is an invitation to treat yourself with care and to redefine what dessert means in your life.

As we move through this collection of healthy desserts, remember that the goal is to enrich your relationship with food, allowing you to indulge in desserts that feel as good to eat as they taste. This is dessert reimagined— where every sweet finish is also a smart start to a healthier, happier you.

9.1 SUGAR-FREE SWEETS TO SATISFY CRAVINGS

In this chapter, we delve into the delightful world of sugar-free sweets that satisfy without the guilt. Recognizing the dietary constraints and health goals of women over 50, these recipes are designed to please the palate without relying on added sugars. Using natural sweeteners like fruits, nuts, and spices, these desserts offer a wonderful alternative to traditional sugary treats, making it possible to indulge your sweet tooth healthily and happily. Each recipe is a testament to the fact that desserts can be both delicious and nourishing, providing the perfect ending to any meal or a sweet snack throughout the day.

ALMOND AND DATE TRUFFLES

PREPARATION TIME: 15 min - **COOKING TIME:** 0 min
MODE OF COOKING: Mixing - **SERVINGS:** 12
INGREDIENTS:
- 1 cup dates, pitted
- 1/2 cup raw almonds
- 1/4 cup unsweetened cocoa powder
- 1 tsp vanilla extract
- 1/4 tsp salt
- Unsweetened shredded coconut, for rolling

DIRECTIONS:
1. In a food processor, blend dates and almonds until they form a sticky paste.
2. Add cocoa powder, vanilla extract, and salt. Pulse until the mixture is well combined.
3. Take small amounts of the mixture and roll into balls.
4. Roll each ball in shredded coconut until well coated.
5. Chill in the refrigerator for at least 1 hour before serving.

TIPS:
- Keep the truffles stored in an airtight container in the refrigerator.
- For a nuttier flavor, roast the almonds before blending.

N.V.: Calories: 100, Fat: 5g, Carbs: 12g, Protein: 2g, Sugar: 9g

AVOCADO CHOCOLATE MOUSSE

PREPARATION TIME: 10 min - **COOKING TIME:** 0 min
MODE OF COOKING: Blending - **SERVINGS:** 4
INGREDIENTS:

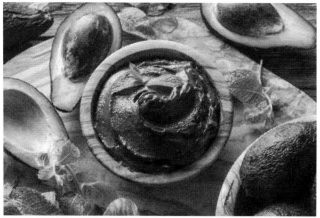

- 2 ripe avocados, peeled and pitted
- 1/4 cup unsweetened cocoa powder
- 1/4 cup almond milk
- 2 Tbsp honey (optional, for strict sugar-free skip this)
- 1 tsp vanilla extract

DIRECTIONS:
1. Combine all ingredients in a blender or food processor.
2. Blend until smooth and creamy.
3. Divide the mousse into serving dishes and refrigerate for at least 1 hour.

TIPS:
- Top with raspberries or a sprinkle of cacao nibs for added texture and flavor.
- If a sweeter taste is desired and honey is not used, consider a sugar-free sweetener like stevia.

N.V.: Calories: 200, Fat: 15g, Carbs: 15g, Protein: 3g, Sugar: 1g

CINNAMON BAKED PEARS

PREPARATION TIME: 5 min - **COOKING TIME:** 25 min
MODE OF COOKING: Baking - **SERVINGS:** 4
INGREDIENTS:

- 4 ripe pears, halved and cored
- 2 Tbsp melted coconut oil
- 2 tsp cinnamon
- 1/4 tsp nutmeg
- 1/4 cup chopped walnuts

DIRECTIONS:
1. Preheat oven to 375°F (190°C).
2. Arrange pear halves cut side up on a baking sheet.
3. Drizzle each pear half with melted coconut oil, then sprinkle with cinnamon and nutmeg.
4. Bake in the preheated oven for 25 minutes, or until pears are soft and slightly golden.
5. Remove from oven, sprinkle with chopped walnuts, and serve warm.

TIPS:
- Serve with a dollop of sugar-free Greek yogurt for added creaminess.
- Experiment with different spices like cloves or cardamom for varied flavors.

N.V.: Calories: 180, Fat: 9g, Carbs: 27g, Protein: 2g, Sugar: 17g (natural sugars from pears)

NO-BAKE PEANUT BUTTER BARS

PREPARATION TIME: 15 min - **COOKING TIME:** 0 min
MODE OF COOKING: Freezing - **SERVINGS:** 8
INGREDIENTS:

- 1 cup natural peanut butter (unsweetened)
- 1/4 cup coconut oil, melted
- 1/4 cup unsweetened shredded coconut
- 1 tsp vanilla extract
- Sugar-free dark chocolate, melted (for drizzling)

DIRECTIONS:
1. Line an 8x8 inch pan with parchment paper.
2. In a medium bowl, mix peanut butter, coconut oil, shredded coconut, and vanilla extract until well combined.
3. Press the mixture evenly into the prepared pan.
4. Drizzle with melted sugar-free dark chocolate.
5. Freeze for at least 2 hours until firm. Cut into bars and serve.

TIPS:
- Keep the bars stored in the freezer to maintain firmness.
- Drizzle with melted sugar-free chocolate before serving for added decadence.

N.V.: Calories: 280, Fat: 24g, Carbs: 8g, Protein: 6g, Sugar: 1g

LEMON CHIA PUDDING

PREPARATION TIME: 10 min (plus chilling) - **COOKING TIME:** 0 min
MODE OF COOKING: Refrigerating - **SERVINGS:** 4
INGREDIENTS:
- 1/4 cup chia seeds
- 1 cup unsweetened almond milk
- Juice and zest of 1 lemon
- 1 tsp vanilla extract
- Sugar-free sweetener to taste (optional)

DIRECTIONS:
1. In a bowl, combine chia seeds, almond milk, lemon juice, lemon zest, and vanilla extract.
2. Whisk thoroughly to combine and prevent clumping.
3. Sweeten to taste, if desired, with a sugar-free sweetener.
4. Cover and refrigerate for at least 4 hours or overnight, until it achieves a pudding-like consistency.

TIPS:
- Top with fresh berries and mint for added freshness and color before serving.
- Adjust the thickness of the pudding by adding more or less almond milk based on your preference.

N.V.: Calories: 120, Fat: 7g, Carbs: 10g, Protein: 4g, Sugar: 0g

9.2 FRESH AND FRUITY TREATS

Celebrating the natural sweetness and vibrant flavors of fruits, this sub-chapter is dedicated to fresh and fruity treats that are both delightful and health-conscious. These recipes harness the goodness of fruits, combining them with other wholesome ingredients to create desserts that are not only indulgent but also nourishing. Perfect for satisfying sweet cravings without overindulgence, each dessert is crafted to bring out the best in seasonal produce, ensuring that every bite is as nutritious as it is delicious. From simple fruit salads to more elaborate concoctions, these desserts are designed to keep you refreshed and satisfied, while aligning with a health-focused lifestyle.

MANGO COCONUT SORBET

PREPARATION TIME: 10 min - **COOKING TIME:** 2 hr (freezing time)
MODE OF COOKING: Freezing - **SERVINGS:** 4
INGREDIENTS:
- 2 ripe mangoes, peeled and cubed
- 1 can (14 oz) coconut milk
- Juice of 1 lime
- 2 Tbsp honey (optional)

DIRECTIONS:
1. Place mango cubes, coconut milk, lime juice, and honey (if using) in a blender. Blend until smooth.
2. Pour the mixture into an ice cream maker and churn according to manufacturer's instructions.
3. Transfer to an airtight container and freeze until firm, about 2 hours.
4. Serve scoops of sorbet garnished with mint leaves or coconut flakes.

TIPS:
- If you do not have an ice cream maker, freeze the mixture in a shallow dish and stir every 30 minutes to break up ice crystals.
- Enhance the tropical flavor by adding a pinch of ground cardamom to the mixture before churning.

N.V.: Calories: 200, Fat: 14g, Carbs: 20g, Protein: 2g, Sugar: 15g

BERRY YOGURT PARFAIT

PREPARATION TIME: 10 min - **COOKING TIME:** 0 min
MODE OF COOKING: Layering - **SERVINGS:** 4
INGREDIENTS:
- 2 cups Greek yogurt
- 1 cup mixed berries (strawberries, blueberries, raspberries)
- 1/4 cup granola
- 2 Tbsp honey or maple syrup (optional)

DIRECTIONS:
1. In serving glasses, layer Greek yogurt, a drizzle of honey or maple syrup, and mixed berries.
2. Repeat the layers until the glasses are filled, ending with berries on top.
3. Garnish with a sprinkle of granola and an extra drizzle of honey or syrup if desired.

TIPS:
- For added texture, include nuts or seeds with the granola.
- Use honey or maple syrup depending on your sweetness preference and dietary needs.

N.V.: Calories: 150, Fat: 2g, Carbs: 21g, Protein: 10g, Sugar: 12g

WATERMELON PIZZA

PREPARATION TIME: 10 min - **COOKING TIME:** 0 min
MODE OF COOKING: Assembly - **SERVINGS:** 4
INGREDIENTS:
- 1 large slice of watermelon, about 1 inch thick, cut from the center to form a round "pizza base"
- 1/4 cup Greek yogurt, spread
- A variety of fresh fruits (kiwi, strawberries, blueberries, grapes), sliced
- A handful of fresh mint, chopped
- Drizzle of honey or a sprinkle of chia seeds (optional)

DIRECTIONS:
1. Lay the watermelon slice on a serving platter.
2. Spread Greek yogurt evenly over the watermelon.
3. Arrange the sliced fruits on top of the yogurt to create "pizza toppings."
4. Garnish with chopped mint and, if desired, a drizzle of honey or a sprinkle of chia seeds for extra flavor and crunch.

TIPS:
- To make this a vegan treat, use coconut yogurt instead of Greek yogurt.
- Chill the watermelon slice before assembling for a refreshing summer dessert.

N.V.: Calories: 120, Fat: 1g, Carbs: 25g, Protein: 4g, Sugar: 18g

CITRUS FRUIT SALAD WITH HONEY LIME DRESSING

PREPARATION TIME: 15 min - **COOKING TIME:** 0 min
MODE OF COOKING: Mixing - **SERVINGS:** 4
INGREDIENTS:
- 1 grapefruit, peeled and sectioned
- 2 oranges, peeled and sectioned
- 2 mandarins, peeled and sectioned
- 1 lime, juice and zest
- 2 Tbsp honey
- Fresh mint leaves, for garnish

DIRECTIONS:
1. In a large bowl, combine grapefruit, oranges, and mandarins.
2. In a small bowl, whisk together lime juice, zest, and honey to create the dressing.
3. Pour the dressing over the citrus fruits and gently toss to coat.
4. Chill in the refrigerator for at least an hour before serving.
5. Garnish with fresh mint leaves just before serving.

TIPS:
- Add pomegranate seeds for a pop of color and texture.
- Serve over a bed of fresh spinach for a healthy, refreshing salad.

N.V.: Calories: 90, Fat: 0g, Carbs: 23g, Protein: 1g, Sugar: 20g

KIWI AND STRAWBERRY LAYERS

PREPARATION TIME: 10 min - **COOKING TIME:** 0 min
MODE OF COOKING: Layering - **SERVINGS:** 4
INGREDIENTS:
- 4 kiwis, peeled and sliced
- 2 cups strawberries, sliced
- 1/2 cup Greek yogurt
- 2 Tbsp honey or maple syrup (optional)
- Fresh mint for garnish

DIRECTIONS:
1. In serving glasses, layer slices of kiwi, a spoonful of Greek yogurt, and slices of strawberries.
2. Repeat the layering process until glasses are filled.
3. Drizzle with honey or maple syrup if desired, and garnish with fresh mint.

TIPS:
- For a crunch, add a layer of granola between the fruits and yogurt.
- Chill the fruits in advance to enhance their freshness and flavor in the dessert.

N.V.: Calories: 120, Fat: 1g, Carbs: 26g, Protein: 3g, Sugar: 18g

9.3 WHOLESOME BAKED GOODS

Embracing the warmth and comfort that only baked goods can offer, this sub-chapter is devoted to wholesome baked desserts that are not only satisfying but also mindful of your health. Each recipe utilizes nutritious ingredients such as whole grains, nuts, seeds, and natural sweeteners to create treats that you can enjoy without guilt. These baked goods are designed to be enjoyed by anyone looking to indulge in a healthier option that doesn't compromise on taste or texture. From moist breads to crispy cookies, these recipes provide a delightful way to conclude a meal or accompany a cozy afternoon tea.

WHOLE WHEAT BANANA BREAD

PREPARATION TIME: 15 min - **COOKING TIME:** 55 min
MODE OF COOKING: Baking - **SERVINGS:** 8
INGREDIENTS:
- 2 cups whole wheat flour
- 4 ripe bananas, mashed
- 1/2 cup unsweetened applesauce
- 1/4 cup honey
- 2 eggs
- 1 tsp baking soda
- 1/2 tsp salt
- 1 tsp vanilla extract
- 1/2 cup walnuts, chopped

DIRECTIONS:
1. Preheat oven to 350°F (175°C). Grease a 9x5 inch loaf pan.
2. In a large bowl, combine flour, baking soda, and salt.
3. In another bowl, mix mashed bananas, applesauce, honey, eggs, and vanilla extract until well blended.
4. Stir banana mixture into the flour mixture until just combined. Fold in walnuts.
5. Pour batter into the prepared loaf pan.
6. Bake in the preheated oven for 55 minutes, or until a toothpick inserted into the center comes out clean.
7. Let bread cool in the pan for 10 minutes, then turn out onto a wire rack.

TIPS:
- Add a sprinkle of cinnamon or nutmeg for a spiced version.
- Replace walnuts with pecans or add dark chocolate chips for a different twist.

N.V.: Calories: 260, Fat: 6g, Carbs: 46g, Protein: 6g, Sugar: 20g

OATMEAL RAISIN COOKIES

PREPARATION TIME: 10 min - **COOKING TIME:** 10 min
MODE OF COOKING: Baking - **SERVINGS:** 12
INGREDIENTS:
- 1 cup rolled oats
- 3/4 cup whole wheat flour
- 1/2 tsp baking soda
- 1/2 tsp cinnamon
- 1/4 tsp salt
- 1/4 cup unsweetened applesauce
- 1/4 cup coconut oil, melted
- 1/2 cup maple syrup
- 1 egg
- 1/2 tsp vanilla extract
- 1/2 cup raisins

DIRECTIONS:
1. Preheat oven to 350°F (175°C). Line a baking sheet with parchment paper.
2. In a bowl, mix oats, flour, baking soda, cinnamon, and salt.
3. In another bowl, whisk together applesauce, coconut oil, maple syrup, egg, and vanilla.
4. Combine the wet and dry ingredients until just mixed, then fold in raisins.
5. Drop tablespoonfuls of dough onto the prepared baking sheet.
6. Bake for 10 minutes, or until edges are golden.
7. Let cookies cool on the baking sheet for 5 minutes before transferring to a wire rack to cool completely.

TIPS:

- Keep cookies in an airtight container to maintain freshness.
- Swap raisins for dried cranberries or add nuts for additional texture.

N.V.: Calories: 160, Fat: 5g, Carbs: 27g, Protein: 3g, Sugar: 12g

CHAPTER 10: DRINKS AND SMOOTHIES

In the golden years of life, as the morning dew refreshes the day, so too can a carefully chosen drink invigorate the body and spirit. Chapter 10 of our journey through intermittent fasting explores the transformative power of drinks and smoothies, designed not just to quench thirst but to enrich your health with every sip. As we navigate the later decades, our bodies crave not only sustenance but also rejuvenation, and what better way to provide this than through the artful blending of flavors and nutrients?

Consider the morning: a time of quiet reflection and the soft ushering in of the day's possibilities. Here, a nutrient-rich smoothie can serve as a gentle wake-up call for your metabolism, infusing your body with vital nutrients without overburdening it. These blends are not merely beverages but morning rituals, crafted to align with the rhythms of a body that has matured like fine wine.

As the day unfolds, the need for hydration and energy becomes paramount, especially when you are aligning your eating schedule with intermittent fasting. This chapter introduces you to a variety of drinks—from herbal teas brimming with antioxidants to smoothies rich in proteins and fibers—that support your fasting goals while tantalizing the palate. Each recipe is a testament to the joy of drinking your way to health, using ingredients that are as beneficial as they are delightful.

Imagine the refreshment of a cool, mint-infused water on a warm afternoon or the creamy luxury of a homemade nut milk smoothie after a morning walk. These drinks do more than satiate; they are crafted to support your body's needs, such as enhancing hydration, boosting metabolic health, and supporting mental clarity.

Join me as we blend, mix, and stir our way to vitality. This chapter isn't just about listing recipes—it's about weaving the essence of these drinks into the fabric of your daily life, making each sip an act of nourishment and a celebration of your health journey. So, raise your glass to the many flavors of health and well-being that await in your new, vibrant fasting lifestyle.

10.1 HERBAL TEAS AND THEIR HEALTH BENEFITS

Herbal teas offer a sanctuary of wellness in every cup, weaving the gentle warmth of tradition with the power of natural healing. In this selection of herbal tea recipes, we explore beverages that not only warm the body but also promote health benefits ranging from improved digestion to enhanced sleep and reduced inflammation. Each recipe is crafted with care, using herbs known for their therapeutic properties. As we delve into these herbal concoctions, we embrace a form of culinary alchemy where every ingredient is purposeful and every sip a step toward better health.

SOOTHING CHAMOMILE MINT TEA

PREPARATION TIME: 5 min - **COOKING TIME:** 10 min
MODE OF COOKING: Simmering - **SERVINGS:** 2
INGREDIENTS:
- 2 Tbsp dried chamomile flowers
- 10 fresh mint leaves
- 2 cups water
- Honey or lemon slices, to taste (optional)

DIRECTIONS:
1. In a small saucepan, bring water to a boil.
2. Add the chamomile flowers and mint leaves to the boiling water and remove from heat.
3. Cover and steep for 10 minutes.
4. Strain the tea into cups, discarding the solids.
5. If desired, sweeten with honey or add a slice of lemon before serving.

TIPS:
- Steeping time can be adjusted based on preferred strength.

- Chamomile is known for its calming effects, making this tea ideal for evening consumption.

N.V.: Calories: 2, Fat: 0g, Carbs: 0.5g, Protein: 0g, Sugar: 0g

GINGER TURMERIC HEALING TEA

PREPARATION TIME: 10 min - **COOKING TIME:** 5 min

MODE OF COOKING: Boiling - **SERVINGS:** 2

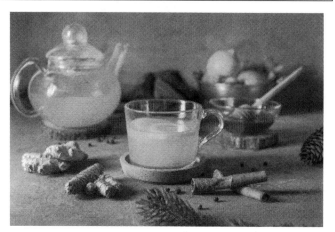

INGREDIENTS:
- 1 inch ginger root, peeled and thinly sliced
- 1 tsp turmeric powder
- 1/2 tsp black pepper (to enhance turmeric absorption)
- 4 cups water
- 1 Tbsp honey, to taste

DIRECTIONS:
1. Combine water, ginger, turmeric, and black pepper in a medium pot and bring to a boil.
2. Reduce heat and simmer for 5 minutes.
3. Strain the mixture into mugs and stir in honey to sweeten.

TIPS:
- Drink warm to maximize benefits, especially during cold weather.
- Ginger and turmeric are powerful anti-inflammatories and antioxidants.

N.V.: Calories: 60, Fat: 0.5g, Carbs: 15g, Protein: 0g, Sugar: 12g

LAVENDER LEMON BALM TEA

PREPARATION TIME: 5 min - **COOKING TIME:** 15 min

MODE OF COOKING: Infusing - **SERVINGS:** 2

INGREDIENTS:
- 1 Tbsp dried lavender flowers
- 1 Tbsp dried lemon balm
- 3 cups boiling water
- Optional: honey or stevia to taste

DIRECTIONS:
1. Place lavender and lemon balm in a tea pot or heatproof pitcher.
2. Pour boiling water over the herbs and cover.
3. Let steep for 15 minutes.
4. Strain the tea and serve hot. Sweeten if desired.

TIPS:
- Lavender is excellent for stress relief, while lemon balm can help ease anxiety.
- For a cooler beverage, chill the tea and serve with ice cubes.

N.V.: Calories: 0, Fat: 0g, Carbs: 0g, Protein: 0g, Sugar: 0g

PEPPERMINT DIGESTIVE TEA

PREPARATION TIME: 5 min - **COOKING TIME:** 10 min

MODE OF COOKING: Steeping - **SERVINGS:** 2

INGREDIENTS:
- 1/4 cup fresh peppermint leaves
- 2 cups water
- Optional: honey or lemon for flavor

DIRECTIONS:
1. Boil water in a kettle.
2. Place peppermint leaves in a teapot or directly into cups.
3. Pour hot water over the leaves and steep for 10 minutes.
4. Strain, then add honey or lemon if using, and serve.

TIPS:
- Peppermint is particularly effective in aiding digestion and relieving stomach aches.
- Can be served hot or cold depending on preference.

N.V.: Calories: 5, Fat: 0g, Carbs: 1g, Protein: 0g, Sugar: 1g

ROSEHIP IMMUNE BOOSTER TEA

PREPARATION TIME: 5 min - **COOKING TIME:** 15 min
MODE OF COOKING: Simmering - **SERVINGS:** 2
INGREDIENTS:
- 2 Tbsp dried rosehip
- 2 cups water
- Optional: cinnamon stick or honey for flavor

DIRECTIONS:
1. In a small saucepan, combine rosehips and water.
2. Bring to a boil, then cover and simmer for 15 minutes.
3. Strain into cups and add a cinnamon stick or honey as desired.

TIPS:
- Rich in vitamin C, rosehips are excellent for strengthening the immune system.
- Serve hot, especially during flu season for added health benefits.

N.V.: Calories: 9, Fat: 0g, Carbs: 2g, Protein: 0g, Sugar: 2g

HIBISCUS REFRESH TEA

PREPARATION TIME: 5 min - **COOKING TIME:** 10 min
MODE OF COOKING: Steeping - **SERVINGS:** 2
INGREDIENTS:
- 1/4 cup dried hibiscus flowers
- 4 cups water
- Ice cubes
- Optional: sweetener of choice

DIRECTIONS:
1. Boil water and pour over the hibiscus flowers in a large pitcher.
2. Allow to steep for 10 minutes.
3. Strain and serve over ice. Sweeten as desired.

TIPS:
- Hibiscus tea is known for its high antioxidants and can help lower blood pressure.
- Its vibrant color makes it a festive choice for gatherings.

N.V.: Calories: 0, Fat: 0g, Carbs: 0g, Protein: 0g, Sugar: 0g

LEMON GINGER DETOX TEA

PREPARATION TIME: 10 min - **COOKING TIME:** 5 min
MODE OF COOKING: Boiling - **SERVINGS:** 2
INGREDIENTS:
- 1 lemon, juiced and zest finely grated
- 1 inch piece of fresh ginger, peeled and sliced
- 2 cups water

- Optional: honey to taste

DIRECTIONS:
1. In a small pot, bring water to a boil. Add ginger and lemon zest, then simmer for 5 minutes.
2. Remove from heat, stir in lemon juice, and strain into cups.
3. Add honey if desired and serve.

TIPS:
- This tea is perfect for cleansing the liver and improving digestion.
- Drink first thing in the morning to kickstart your metabolism.

N.V.: Calories: 10, Fat: 0g, Carbs: 3g, Protein: 0g, Sugar: 2g

10.2 DETOXIFYING JUICES AND SMOOTHIES

Embarking on a journey to purify your body and invigorate your spirit with nourishing liquids, this section unfolds a series of detoxifying juices and smoothies. Each concoction is designed to cleanse your system, boost your metabolism, and enhance your energy levels, all while delivering essential nutrients in delicious liquid form. From vibrant vegetable blends to sweet, antioxidant-rich fruit mixes, these drinks are more than just refreshing—they are a cornerstone of a healthful approach to living that supports your body's natural detox processes. Let's explore how these nutrient-dense beverages can become a vital part of your daily routine, promoting a clearer, brighter, and more energetic lifestyle.

GREEN DETOX SMOOTHIE

PREPARATION TIME: 10 min - **COOKING TIME:** 0 min
MODE OF COOKING: Blending - **SERVINGS:** 1
INGREDIENTS:
- 1 cup spinach leaves
- 1 small cucumber, chopped
- 1 green apple, cored and sliced
- 1/2 lemon, juiced
- 1 Tbsp chia seeds
- 1 cup coconut water

DIRECTIONS:
1. Place all ingredients in a blender.
2. Blend on high until smooth and creamy.
3. Serve immediately.

TIPS:
- Add a piece of ginger for an extra kick and digestive benefits.
- Ensure the smoothie is consumed immediately to retain all nutrients.

N.V.: Calories: 180, Fat: 1g, Carbs: 40g, Protein: 3g, Sugar: 30g

---

BEETROOT AND GINGER JUICE

PREPARATION TIME: 10 min - **COOKING TIME:** 0 min
MODE OF COOKING: Juicing - **SERVINGS:** 2
INGREDIENTS:
- 2 medium beetroots, peeled and diced
- 1 inch ginger root
- 2 carrots, peeled and diced
- 1/2 lemon, juiced
- 1 apple, cored and sliced

DIRECTIONS:
1. Feed all ingredients except lemon juice through a juicer.

2. Stir in the lemon juice after juicing.
3. Serve chilled.

TIPS:
- Drink immediately to maximize the benefits of enzymes and nutrients.
- Add a pinch of cayenne pepper for an extra detoxifying effect.

N.V.: Calories: 120, Fat: 0.5g, Carbs: 29g, Protein: 2g, Sugar: 21g

CARROT LIVER FLUSH

PREPARATION TIME: 8 min - **COOKING TIME:** 0 min
MODE OF COOKING: Juicing - **SERVINGS:** 1
INGREDIENTS:
- 4 large carrots
- 1/2 beetroot, peeled
- 2 stalks celery
- 1/2 lemon, juiced
- 1 Tbsp olive oil

DIRECTIONS:
1. Juice carrots, beetroot, and celery.
2. Mix in the lemon juice and olive oil.
3. Serve immediately for best flavor and health benefits.

TIPS:
- Olive oil helps absorb the soluble vitamins in the juice.
- Ideal for a morning detox routine.

N.V.: Calories: 140, Fat: 14g, Carbs: 15g, Protein: 2g, Sugar: 9g

SPICY LEMONADE CLEANSE

PREPARATION TIME: 5 min - **COOKING TIME:** 0 min
MODE OF COOKING: Mixing - **SERVINGS:** 1
INGREDIENTS:
- 2 cups filtered water
- Juice of 1 lemon
- 1 Tbsp maple syrup
- 1/10 tsp cayenne pepper

DIRECTIONS:
1. Combine all ingredients in a large glass.
2. Stir well until the maple syrup is fully dissolved.
3. Serve chilled or at room temperature.

TIPS:
- Adjust the amount of cayenne pepper according to tolerance and preference.
- This drink is excellent for boosting metabolism.

N.V.: Calories: 50, Fat: 0g, Carbs: 14g, Protein: 0g, Sugar: 12g

TROPICAL TURMERIC CLEANSE

PREPARATION TIME: 10 min - **COOKING TIME:** 0 min
MODE OF COOKING: Blending - **SERVINGS:** 2
INGREDIENTS:
- 1 cup pineapple chunks
- 1 mango, peeled and diced
- 1/2 tsp turmeric powder
- 1 cup coconut water

- Juice of 1/2 lime

DIRECTIONS:
1. Place all ingredients in a blender.
2. Blend until smooth.
3. Serve immediately to ensure potency of nutrients.

TIPS:
- Ideal for an anti-inflammatory boost and digestion aid.
- Add a tablespoon of flaxseeds for extra fiber.

N.V.: Calories: 150, Fat: 1g, Carbs: 35g, Protein: 2g, Sugar: 30g

CUCUMBER MINT REFRESH

PREPARATION TIME: 7 min - **COOKING TIME:** 0 min
MODE OF COOKING: Blending - **SERVINGS:** 1
INGREDIENTS:
- 1 large cucumber, chopped
- 10 mint leaves
- Juice of 1 lime
- 1/2 cup water
- Ice cubes

DIRECTIONS:
1. Blend cucumber, mint leaves, lime juice, and water until smooth.
2. Serve over ice.

TIPS:
- Perfect for hydration and cooling down on a hot day.
- Enhance with a splash of club soda for a fizzy variant.

N.V.: Calories: 50, Fat: 0.5g, Carbs: 12g, Protein: 2g, Sugar: 6g

ANTIOXIDANT BERRY BLAST

PREPARATION TIME: 10 min - **COOKING TIME:** 0 min
MODE OF COOKING: Blending - **SERVINGS:** 2
INGREDIENTS:
- 1/2 cup blueberries
- 1/2 cup raspberries
- 1/2 cup strawberries
- 1 cup almond milk
- 1 Tbsp chia seeds

DIRECTIONS:
1. Combine all ingredients in a blender.
2. Blend until smooth.
3. Serve immediately to preserve antioxidants.

TIPS:
- Serve as a nutritious breakfast or a refreshing snack.
- Top with a sprinkle of granola for a crunch.

N.V.: Calories: 130, Fat: 4g, Carbs: 22g, Protein: 3g, Sugar: 12g

10.3 HOMEMADE NUT MILK AND MORE

In the quest for wholesome, nutrient-rich alternatives to conventional dairy, homemade nut milks and other plant-based drinks stand out as both a delightful and nourishing option. This section delves into the art of crafting your own beverages from the simplest of ingredients—nuts, seeds, and grains—transforming them into creamy, flavorful milks and more. Each recipe not only offers a dairy-free delight but also ensures that you're sipping on drinks free from preservatives and artificial additives. Embrace the satisfying process of creating these staples in your own kitchen, enjoying their fresh, natural taste and the health benefits they bring.

CLASSIC ALMOND MILK

PREPARATION TIME: 10 min + soaking overnight
COOKING TIME: 0 min
MODE OF COOKING: Blending
SERVINGS: 4
INGREDIENTS:
- 1 cup raw almonds, soaked overnight
- 4 cups filtered water
- 1 Tbsp vanilla extract
- 2 Tbsp maple syrup (optional)
- Pinch of salt

DIRECTIONS:
1. Drain and rinse the almonds after soaking them overnight.
2. Combine the almonds and filtered water in a blender. Blend on high speed until smooth, about 2 minutes.
3. Over a large bowl, pour the mixture through a nut milk bag or fine mesh strainer to separate the pulp.
4. Return the strained milk to the blender, add vanilla, maple syrup, and salt, and blend to mix.
5. Store in the refrigerator and shake well before serving.

TIPS:
- The leftover almond pulp can be used for baking or as a fiber-rich addition to oatmeal.
- For a sweeter flavor, adjust the amount of maple syrup to taste.

N.V.: Calories: 60, Fat: 4g, Carbs: 2g, Protein: 2g, Sugar: 1g

CREAMY CASHEW MILK

PREPARATION TIME: 10 min + soaking for 2 hrs
COOKING TIME: 0 min
MODE OF COOKING: Blending
SERVINGS: 4
INGREDIENTS:
- 1 cup raw cashews, soaked for 2 hours
- 4 cups water
- 1 tsp vanilla extract
- 1 Tbsp honey or agave syrup (optional)

DIRECTIONS:
1. Drain and rinse the soaked cashews thoroughly.
2. Place cashews, water, vanilla extract, and sweetener (if using) in a blender. Blend on high until completely smooth.
3. Strain through a nut milk bag to remove any grit (optional).
4. Store the cashew milk in a sealed container in the refrigerator.

TIPS:
- Soaking cashews for more than 2 hours can create an even creamier milk.
- Add a pinch of cinnamon or nutmeg for a spiced version.

N.V.: Calories: 90, Fat: 6g, Carbs: 6g, Protein: 3g, Sugar: 2g

SUNFLOWER SEED MILK

PREPARATION TIME: 10 min + soaking overnight
COOKING TIME: 0 min
MODE OF COOKING: Blending
SERVINGS: 4
INGREDIENTS:

- 1 cup raw sunflower seeds, soaked overnight
- 4 cups water
- 1 Tbsp honey or maple syrup
- 1/2 tsp vanilla extract

DIRECTIONS:

1. Drain and rinse the soaked sunflower seeds.
2. Combine seeds with water, sweetener, and vanilla in a blender. Blend until smooth.
3. Strain the mixture using a nut milk bag to remove any remaining solids.
4. Refrigerate and shake before use.

TIPS:

- This milk can be a base for smoothies or as a dairy-free option for coffee.
- Sunflower seed milk is naturally high in Vitamin E, beneficial for skin health.

N.V.: Calories: 70, Fat: 5g, Carbs: 4g, Protein: 2g, Sugar: 3g

WEEK 1	breakfast	snack	lunch	snack	dinner
Monday	Antioxidant Berry Flax Smoothie	Almond Butter Banana Bites	Super Greens Antioxidant Salad	Oat and Berry Energy Bars	Lemon Herb Baked Salmon
Tuesday	Green Detox Smoothie	Greek Yogurt Fruit Cups	Beetroot and Quinoa Antioxidant	Chickpea and Avocado Toast	Stuffed Chicken Parmesan
Wednesday	Zucchini and Parmesan Breakfast	Spinach and Cheese Egg Muffins	Turkey and Avocado Wrap	Sweet Potato Hummus	Cauliflower Risotto with Shrimp
Thursday	Almond Joy Overnight Oats	Apple Peanut Butter Sandwiches	Chicken Caesar Salad Wrap	Cottage Cheese and Fruit Plate	Beef and Broccoli Stir-Fry
Friday	Sun-dried Tomato and Spinach	High Protein Cottage Cheese	Curried Chicken Salad Wrap	Oatmeal and Chia Seed Pudding	Portobello Mushroom Pizza
Saturday	Nutrient-Rich Smoothies	Smoked Salmon and Cream Cheese	Grilled Vegetable and Goat	Avocado and Shrimp Salad	Roasted Tomato and Basil Soup
Sunday	Sweet Potato and Black Bean	Mediterranean Vegetable Wrap	Tuna and White Bean Salad Wrap	Roasted Chickpeas	Pumpkin Ginger Soup

WEEK 2	breakfast	snack	lunch	snack	dinner
Monday	Savory Mushroom and Spinach	Greek Yogurt Fruit Cups	Turkey and Avocado Wrap	Chickpea and Avocado Toast	Stuffed Chicken Parmesan
Tuesday	Cottage Cheese and Chive	Almond Butter Banana Bites	Curried Chicken Salad Wrap	Oatmeal and Chia Seed Pudding	Beef and Broccoli Stir-Fry
Wednesday	Almond Joy Overnight Oats	Apple Peanut Butter Sandwiches	Grilled Vegetable and Goat	Sweet Potato Hummus	Cauliflower Risotto with Shrimp
Thursday	Zucchini and Parmesan Breakfast	Spinach and Cheese Egg Muffins	Mediterranean Vegetable Wrap	Avocado and Shrimp Salad	Portobello Mushroom Pizza
Friday	Sun-dried Tomato and Spinach	Smoked Salmon and Cream Cheese	Chicken Caesar Salad Wrap	Cottage Cheese and Fruit Plate	Roasted Tomato and Basil Soup
Saturday	Nutrient-Rich Smoothies	High Protein Cottage Cheese	Tuna and White Bean Salad Wrap	Roasted Chickpeas	Lemon Herb Baked Salmon
Sunday	Sweet Potato and Black Bean	Oat and Berry Energy Bars	Beetroot and Quinoa Antioxidant	Chickpea and Avocado Toast	Pumpkin Ginger Soup

WEEK 3	breakfast	snack	lunch	snack	dinner
Monday	Cottage Cheese and Chive	Greek Yogurt Fruit Cups	Curried Chicken Salad Wrap	Chickpea and Avocado Toast	Stuffed Chicken Parmesan
Tuesday	Savory Mushroom and Spinach	Almond Butter Banana Bites	Tuna and White Bean Salad Wrap	Sweet Potato Hummus	Beef and Broccoli Stir-Fry
Wednesday	Smoked Salmon and Avocado	Apple Peanut Butter Sandwiches	Mediterranean Vegetable Wrap	Oatmeal and Chia Seed Pudding	Cauliflower Risotto with Shrimp
Thursday	Sun-dried Tomato and Spinach	High Protein Cottage Cheese	Grilled Vegetable and Goat	Roasted Chickpeas	Pumpkin Ginger Soup
Friday	Almond Joy Overnight Oats	Spinach and Cheese Egg Muffins	Chicken Caesar Salad Wrap	Cottage Cheese and Fruit Plate	Roasted Tomato and Basil Soup
Saturday	Zucchini and Parmesan Breakfast	Smoked Salmon and Cream Cheese	Turkey and Avocado Wrap	Avocado and Shrimp Salad	Lemon Herb Baked Salmon
Sunday	Nutrient-Rich Smoothies	Oat and Berry Energy Bars	Beetroot and Quinoa Antioxidant	Greek Yogurt Fruit Cups	Portobello Mushroom Pizza

WEEK 4	breakfast	snack	lunch	snack	dinner
Monday	Zucchini and Parmesan Breakfast	Greek Yogurt Fruit Cups	Turkey and Avocado Wrap	Chickpea and Avocado Toast	Stuffed Chicken Parmesan
Tuesday	Cottage Cheese and Chive	Almond Butter Banana Bites	Curried Chicken Salad Wrap	Oatmeal and Chia Seed Pudding	Beef and Broccoli Stir-Fry
Wednesday	Savory Mushroom and Spinach	Apple Peanut Butter Sandwiches	Grilled Vegetable and Goat	Sweet Potato Hummus	Cauliflower Risotto with Shrimp
Thursday	Almond Joy Overnight Oats	Spinach and Cheese Egg Muffins	Mediterranean Vegetable Wrap	Avocado and Shrimp Salad	Pumpkin Ginger Soup
Friday	Sun-dried Tomato and Spinach	Smoked Salmon and Cream Cheese	Chicken Caesar Salad Wrap	Cottage Cheese and Fruit Plate	Lemon Herb Baked Salmon
Saturday	Sweet Potato and Black Bean	Oat and Berry Energy Bars	Beetroot and Quinoa Antioxidant	Greek Yogurt Fruit Cups	Portobello Mushroom Pizza
Sunday	Nutrient-Rich Smoothies	High Protein Cottage Cheese	Tuna and White Bean Salad Wrap	Roasted Chickpeas	Roasted Tomato and Basil Soup

CHAPTER 11: INTERMITTENT FASTING SUCCESS STRATEGIES

Embracing intermittent fasting is akin to learning a new dance. It's about finding a rhythm that suits your life's melody and the subtle changes in tempo that come with the years. In this chapter, we delve into the strategies that can make intermittent fasting not just an experiment, but a successful and sustainable part of your lifestyle. It's about transforming knowledge into practice, and practice into a routine that feels as natural as breathing.

The journey of intermittent fasting is both personal and profound. It asks you to listen intently to the needs of your body, to understand its cues, and to respond with care. This chapter is your guide through that process. It doesn't merely recount the steps but illuminates the pathway so you can navigate the highs and lows with confidence. Here, we explore how to align your fasting protocol with your body's natural rhythms, enhancing your metabolic health and enriching your life with vitality.

Success in intermittent fasting doesn't come from rigid adherence to rules but from adapting the principles to fit your individual circumstances. This approach helps manage everything from appetite to energy levels, ensuring that each day you are nourished and none of the joy of eating is lost. We'll share insights on how to start your fasting journey, how to overcome the common hurdles, and how to measure your progress in ways that encourage persistence and adjustment.

Moreover, this chapter addresses the importance of mental and emotional preparation as you adapt to a new way of eating. Understanding that occasional setbacks are part of the journey helps fortify your resolve and keeps you focused on the long-term benefits. With each section, you'll find practical tips that are easy to integrate into your daily routine, ensuring that intermittent fasting becomes a seamless part of your quest for health without overwhelming your day-to-day life.

By the end of this chapter, intermittent fasting will feel less like a dietary challenge and more like a rewarding lifestyle that you are well-equipped to maintain. It's about making empowered choices that support your health goals while still enjoying life's culinary pleasures.

11.1 TRACKING YOUR PROGRESS EFFECTIVELY

Embarking on the intermittent fasting journey is akin to setting out on a new adventure where each step, turn, and discovery is vital to understanding and mastering the terrain. To navigate this path successfully, one of the most crucial tools at your disposal is the ability to track your progress effectively. This isn't merely about marking days on a calendar or celebrating weight milestones; it's about deepening your understanding of how your body responds to various fasting schedules and dietary adjustments, and refining your approach based on real, tangible data.

The Art of Self-Observation

At its core, effective progress tracking in intermittent fasting involves a blend of quantitative and qualitative measures. Quantitatively, you might track weight, body measurements, and perhaps more clinical metrics like blood pressure or glucose levels if you're managing specific health conditions. Qualitatively, it's essential to assess your energy levels, hunger patterns, emotional state, and overall well-being.

This dual approach allows you to see not just the physical changes that occur with intermittent fasting but also the subtle shifts in your mental and emotional landscape. It's about capturing the full spectrum of your health evolution, painting a comprehensive picture that guides your decisions and modifications to your fasting regimen.

Tools for Tracking

In the digital age, numerous tools can assist in monitoring your intermittent fasting progress. Mobile apps specifically designed for fasting provide timers, reminders, and sometimes integration with fitness trackers to monitor your activity levels and physiological changes. These apps often include features for logging meals and noting how you feel at various points in your fasting cycle, making them invaluable for spotting trends and triggers.

Journaling is another powerful tool, especially for the qualitative side of tracking. Regular entries about your fasting experience can help you identify patterns that affect your mood, energy, and hunger levels. For instance, you may notice that certain foods consumed during your eating window influence your ease of fasting the following day, or that your mental clarity improves significantly after several weeks of consistent fasting.

Understanding Weight Fluctuations

Weight is often the most common metric people use to gauge the success of their fasting efforts. However, it's crucial to approach weight tracking with a nuanced perspective. Weight can fluctuate due to a variety of factors including water retention, muscle gain, and the time of day. Thus, weighing yourself at the same time and under the same conditions—preferably in the morning before eating or drinking—can provide a more accurate reflection of your true weight changes.

Moreover, focusing solely on the scale can be misleading. Incorporating body measurements such as waist, hips, and even neck circumference can provide more insights into how your body composition is changing, potentially showing you a decrease in body fat even when your weight remains constant.

The Role of Feedback Loops

As you gather data on your fasting journey, the concept of feedback loops becomes incredibly relevant. This involves using the information you collect to make informed adjustments to your fasting plan. For example, if you consistently note a slump in energy in the late afternoon, you might experiment with shifting your eating window or altering its contents to include more slow-releasing energy sources like complex carbohydrates or healthy fats.

Feedback loops also help in setting realistic goals and expectations. By understanding your body's responses, you can better predict how it might react to different fasting durations or schedules, and set achievable targets that propel you forward without causing burnout or disappointment.

Psychological and Social Considerations

Tracking your progress in intermittent fasting is not just about observing what happens when you're alone; it's also about understanding how your social interactions and emotional states influence your fasting success. Social engagements, for example, can pose challenges to maintaining your fasting window, and tracking how you handle these situations can provide insights into when and how to schedule your fasting periods.

Emotionally, how you feel about your progress can affect your motivation and commitment. Regularly assessing your satisfaction with the process and the outcomes can help you maintain a positive and constructive attitude towards fasting. It's important to celebrate the small victories along the way—perhaps a newfound ability to resist cravings or the completion of a particularly challenging fasting period.

Long-term Trends and Health Outcomes

Finally, tracking your progress effectively in intermittent fasting should always be aimed at long-term health enhancement. Short-term gains are encouraging, but the true benefits of intermittent fasting often show over longer periods. Chronic diseases, longevity, and overall life quality are profoundly impacted by dietary habits, and fasting can be a pivotal factor in improving these aspects of health.

As you compile data over months or even years, patterns will emerge that provide deep insights into the best ways to sustain and optimize your health through fasting. This long-view approach not only ensures that intermittent fasting remains a viable and beneficial part of your lifestyle but also helps in continuously aligning the practice with your evolving health needs and life circumstances.

By effectively tracking your progress, you arm yourself with knowledge—not just about fasting, but about your body's unique responses, empowering you to make informed, health-promoting decisions that resonate deeply with your personal health journey.

11.2 Tips for Staying Motivated

Embarking on the journey of intermittent fasting can feel like steering a ship through uncharted waters. It requires dedication, adaptability, and above all, sustained motivation. Motivation is not merely a spark but a continuous flame that must be nurtured and fed, especially when navigating the transformative yet challenging waters of lifestyle change. Here, we delve into the essence of staying motivated, unpacking strategies that resonate deeply with the experiences of many who have ventured down this path.

Building a Vision

Motivation thrives on vision. Start by clearly defining why you are adopting intermittent fasting. Is it to improve your metabolic health, extend your longevity, manage weight, or perhaps enhance mental clarity? Understanding your 'why' anchors your motivation, turning it into a beacon that guides your daily choices. Create a vision board or a journal dedicated to your fasting journey. Populate it with images, quotes, and affirmations that align with your health goals, turning to it whenever you feel your resolve wavering.

Setting Achievable Goals

While lofty goals can feel inspiring, they can also be daunting. Break your ultimate objective into smaller, manageable goals. Celebrate each milestone, whether it's completing your first full week of fasting, reaching a certain weight, or simply feeling more energetic. These victories provide a steady stream of encouragement, each one propelling you closer to your larger goal.

Cultivating a Supportive Community

The path of intermittent fasting can be lonely if trodden alone. Surround yourself with a community of like-minded individuals who are on similar journeys. This could be through online forums, local health groups, or even friends and family members who share your interest in health and wellness. Regular discussions and check-ins can keep you accountable and offer a platform for sharing challenges and successes.

Integrating Flexibility in Your Approach

Rigidity can be the downfall of motivation. Life's unpredictability means that your fasting schedule might need occasional adjustments. Rather than viewing these adjustments as failures, treat them as informed decisions that cater to your body's needs. This flexible approach helps maintain motivation, making the fasting lifestyle sustainable rather than a sporadic sprint.

Leveraging Technology

In today's digital age, numerous apps and tools can help keep you on track. Use apps that not only track your fasting and feeding windows but also provide motivational reminders and educational content. This technology can serve as both a tracker and a coach, keeping you informed and inspired.

Maintaining Nutritional Balance

A common demotivator is the feeling of deprivation. Ensure that your eating windows are filled with nutrient-dense and satisfying foods. A well-nourished body supports a well-motivated mind. When your body feels good, your mind is more likely to remain committed. Explore new recipes and foods that bring excitement to your meals, making each eating window something to look forward to.

Embracing Educational Growth

Understand the science behind intermittent fasting. Knowledge is motivational, especially when it connects what you are doing with why you are doing it. Read up on the latest research, watch documentaries, and attend seminars. This continuous learning process can reignite your motivation by reminding you of the tangible benefits of intermittent fasting.

Reflecting on the Journey

Regular reflection can significantly boost motivation. Take time to reflect on your journey—what's been working, what hasn't, and how you feel both physically and mentally. Writing down these reflections can be particularly powerful, offering insights that drive deeper commitment.

Managing Stress Effectively

Stress can erode motivation, making even the best-laid plans feel burdensome. Incorporate stress management techniques such as meditation, yoga, or even simple breathing exercises into your routine. Reducing stress not only helps maintain motivation but also enhances the overall benefits of intermittent fasting.

Visualizing Success

Visualization is a potent tool in maintaining motivation. Regularly spend a few minutes visualizing yourself achieving your goals. See yourself healthier, more energetic, and thriving. This mental imagery can boost your emotional and psychological motivation, keeping you firmly on the path.

Celebrating the Non-Scale Victories

Finally, remember that motivation often comes from recognizing changes that aren't always reflected on the scale. Maybe you have more energy, better skin, improved sleep, or a sharper mind. Celebrate these non-scale victories as they often provide the most meaningful motivation to continue.

Motivation in the realm of intermittent fasting is not just about willpower but about weaving a tapestry of strategies that resonate with your lifestyle, goals, and personal growth. It's about crafting a journey that is as rewarding as the destination itself. With each day, with each choice, you are not just fasting; you are curating a lifestyle that aligns with your vision of health and vitality.

11.3 ADJUSTING YOUR DIET AS YOU AGE

As the chapters of our lives unfold, our bodies and nutritional needs undergo a series of evolutions. Intermittent fasting, when practiced during the golden years, requires adjustments to complement the shifting landscape of our physical health. Understanding and embracing these changes ensures that intermittent fasting remains a beneficial and sustainable lifestyle choice as you age.

The Evolving Body

With age, our metabolism naturally slows down, muscle mass tends to decrease, and many experience changes in digestive efficiency and hormonal balance. These shifts necessitate adjustments in dietary intake to support continued health and vitality. The beauty of intermittent fasting is its adaptability; it can evolve with you, accommodating your body's changing needs.

Nutritional Needs and Aging

As you grow older, your body becomes less efficient at absorbing certain nutrients, increasing the risk of deficiencies in vitamins such as B12, D, and minerals like calcium and magnesium. It's crucial to focus on nutrient-dense foods during your eating windows to counteract these inefficiencies. Foods rich in fiber, protein, and healthy fats should become staples to help maintain muscle mass, support heart health, and ensure you feel full and satisfied.

Adjusting Fasting Windows

One size does not fit all, especially as you age. You may find that shorter fasting periods are more suitable as they can be easier on the body and still provide significant health benefits. For instance, shifting from a 16-hour fast to a 14-hour or even 12-hour fast can help maintain energy levels and support more regular nutrient intake, crucial for older adults.

Listening to Your Body

As you age, listening to your body becomes more crucial than ever. If you experience fatigue, dizziness, or other adverse symptoms, it may be necessary to adjust your fasting protocol. This could mean altering the length of your fasting window, the timing of your meals, or even the composition of your meals to ensure that your body is adequately nourished.

Hydration and Electrolyte Balance

Hydration is vital at any age, but it becomes even more crucial as you grow older. The body's ability to conserve water decreases with age, and the sense of thirst may not be as acute. Ensuring adequate hydration during fasting and non-fasting periods is essential. Additionally, maintaining a balance of electrolytes like sodium, potassium, and magnesium can help prevent dehydration and support overall cellular function.

Incorporating Physical Activity

Maintaining an active lifestyle complements the benefits of intermittent fasting. As you age, consider integrating gentle, regular physical activities such as walking, yoga, or swimming, which support muscle health and mobility without overly taxing the body. Exercise, coupled with fasting, can help regulate blood sugar levels, enhance mental health, and boost overall energy levels.

Regular Medical Consultations

Regular check-ups with your healthcare provider are essential to safely manage intermittent fasting as you age. Medical guidance is invaluable, especially when adjusting your diet or fasting schedule to accommodate health conditions like diabetes, hypertension, or heart disease. Always consult a healthcare professional before making significant changes to your fasting routine, particularly if you are taking medications or managing chronic illnesses.

Mental and Emotional Health

Adjusting your diet as you age is not solely about physical health; it's also about nurturing your mental and emotional well-being. Intermittent fasting can enhance brain health by improving mood and cognitive function.

However, it's important to approach fasting with a mindset that values flexibility and self-compassion, recognizing that your dietary needs and abilities may change over time.

Social Engagements and Lifestyle

Dining and socializing play significant roles in our lives, especially as we age. Adjusting your intermittent fasting schedule to accommodate social interactions can help maintain a balanced, enjoyable lifestyle. This might mean planning your fasting windows around family gatherings or social outings, ensuring that your dietary regimen enhances your social life rather than constraining it.

Long-Term Sustainability

Ultimately, the goal of adjusting your diet as you age is to ensure the long-term sustainability of intermittent fasting. This means continuously adapting and refining your approach to meet your body's needs, supporting a lifestyle that enhances your quality of life and longevity. By being proactive about these adjustments, intermittent fasting can continue to be a valuable part of your wellness routine, providing benefits that extend well into your later years.

Embracing the dynamic nature of our bodies as we age requires a thoughtful, informed approach to intermittent fasting. By adjusting and adapting, you can ensure that this powerful health strategy continues to serve you well, enhancing your vitality and well-being throughout all life's stages.

Made in United States
Orlando, FL
18 December 2024

55988650R00061